Dysphagia and Nutrition

Antonio Amitrano

Dysphagia and Nutrition

The Meal of a Patient with Swallowing Disorders

Springer

Antonio Amitrano
Speech Therapist
Rome, Italy

ISBN 978-3-031-77451-5 ISBN 978-3-031-77449-2 (eBook)
https://doi.org/10.1007/978-3-031-77449-2

The original submitted manuscript has been translated into English. The translation was done using artificial intelligence. A subsequent revision was performed by the author(s) to further refine the work and to ensure that the translation is appropriate concerning content and scientific correctness. It may, however, read stylistically different from a conventional translation.

This Springer imprint is published by the registered company Springer Nature Switzerland AG
The registered company address is: Gewerbestrasse 11, 6330 Cham, Switzerland

To Mario, Matilde, Stefano, and Giacomo

My last arrows shot into the future

Foreword

Once again, in this further editorial effort, Antonio Amitrano demonstrates his ability to argue about a human function—now the case of swallowing—not only with the scientific rigor of the health professional but also with the curiosity of someone who seeks to understand and explain the reasoning behind the various customs that accompany this function and, last but not least, with the humanity of those who address not only the patient but also the individual—whether man, woman, or child—deprived of the joy that sitting at the table to eat can bestow.

This multifaceted approach has already characterized *The Voice: A Tool of Professionals Who Promote Health*, a book published in 2004, which I had read with enthusiasm, fascinated by the 1000 facets in which the voice was reflected and analyzed.

In *Dysphagia and Nutrition: The Meal of a Patient with Swallowing Disorders,* the same apparatus that, in the most recent phylogenetic evolution, has allowed people to communicate with voice and speech, is analyzed in terms of its primordial and vital functions, ensuring the supply of nutrients and the defense of the respiratory tract.

The first part of the volume, enriched by numerous anecdotes and historical and cultural references, describes everything that the meal has represented and represents for the human being in terms of sharing, sociability, and joy of living. This first part is a necessary premise, even if previously neglected in other texts, to understand the importance of focusing all efforts on fully recovering oral feeding (per os) in pathological cases or, if not possible, making swallowing "functional," or possible with some tricks, as pleasant and rewarding as possible, thus transforming it into a moment of pleasure and sociability.

The second part of this book describes in detail the physiology and pathophysiology of swallowing and the diagnostic and rehabilitative path that patients with swallowing disorders must undergo. As far as the discussion follows the traditional canons of deglutology doctrine, there are references to tests and techniques recently introduced. Of particular interest is the description of diagnostic methods, such as meal observation, the result of the author's long field experience.

Over the past 30 years, interest in swallowing disorders has spread to involve most health professionals, particularly those who carry out their activities in hospitals and residential facilities for elderly individuals. I believe that reading this volume can offer each of them not only useful technical knowledge to safeguard the health of patients but also essential food for thought, encouraging consideration of feeding problems also from the patient's perspective, thus adopting a broader view that is necessary to optimize therapeutic intervention.

Phoniatric- University of Rome "La Sapienza"
Rome, Italy
Giovanni Ruoppolo

Introduction

The meal, from the Latin *pastus*, is the time dedicated to the intake of food. The distribution of meals throughout the day and the way they are consumed, even though globalization tends to flatten their peculiarities, is significantly different in various geographical regions and different cultures. Despite the diversity present in various geographical areas, "meal" universally refers to the time when food is consumed.

The subtitle of the volume, *The Meal of a Patient With a Swallowing Disorder*, apparently expresses a paradox. The meal, in fact, is based on the consumption of food and therefore on eating. To eat, which introduces food into the digestive system, humans use swallowing, a complex function that ensures the passage of food from the outside to the inside of the body. In some subjects, the ability to swallow is variously compromised by the presence of dysphagia, which in fact determines the difficulty or impossibility of swallowing and therefore of consuming food.

Dysphagia is a symptom present in many individuals with neurological diseases, in individuals undergoing surgical interventions in the head–neck district, and in elderly individuals. Epidemiological studies indicate that approximately 22% of subjects over 50 years of age suffer from some form of dysphagia, whereas the percentage increases to 40% for subjects over 60 years of age. In the world population, the percentage of people over 60 has risen from 9.2% in 1990 to 11.7% in 2013 and is estimated to grow to 21.1% by 2050. The World Health Organization has classified dysphagia in the *International Statistical Classification of Diseases and Related Health Problems* (ICD-9 and ICD-10) (787.2, R13). *Symptom* dysphagia can present with various levels of severity, ranging from an impediment to consuming certain textures to the total inability to take food orally. Dysphagia results in significant consequences, such as aspiration pneumonia, malnutrition, and dehydration, a reduction in quality of life, and death.

Aspiration pneumonia is one of the main consequences of dysphagia, and the WHO indicated that it was the fourth cause of death worldwide in the course of the year 2012. Pneumonia also contributes to increasing the hospitalization rate, particularly in the elderly population. The gap between morbidity and mortality for dysphagia worldwide is significant, as are the costs associated with related nutritional and respiratory complications and the resources used in its management.

In the most severe form of dysphagia, the subject is fed through tubes that directly reach the digestive system and ensure nutrition in times and ways that are no longer those of the meal. The infusion of nutrients takes place over a long period, using several hours of the day or the entire night. The meal is no longer a shared moment and no longer takes place at the table. The subject is in a sitting or semireclining position, in bed or in a chair, connected with a catheter to an infusion pump that slowly transfers the contents of the nutritional mixture bag to the digestive system. In less severe forms of dysphagia, patients manage to eat orally, although with limitations, through the use of strategies that increase the degree of meal safety: very often, they consume their meals in solitude and in places different from those used by the family group to which they belong. The purpose of the volume is to examine how a meal can continue to be an important moment in daily life, even for dysphagic individuals. At the same time, it illustrates the management and safety aspects that can make meals accessible to patients with the supervision of trained caregivers. In fact, it occupies an important part of everyone's life, both in terms of the total time employees spend and the social role they play. Eating in the company of others represents a moment of social interaction and a place where relationships and friendships are strengthened, as well as business and alliances. For dysphagic patients, it is therefore important to preserve this essential moment of social life. Moreover, even in situations extremely compromised from a deglutological point of view, it is appropriate to identify ways to allow food to continue to be the source of pleasure that greatly affects a person's quality of life while respecting safety criteria. Therefore, we analyze various situations of chronic dysphagia in which, with due caution, it is appropriate to find solutions that allow patients who are now deprived of oral feeding, to continue to experience the pleasure of savoring their favorite dishes. The concept of *palliative feeding* must become part of the daily activity of operators assisting patients with severe and irreversible dysphagia and terminally ill patients. If the goal of *palliative medicine* is to improve, as much as possible, the quality of life of subjects who are no longer curable, attention to nutrition must fully fall within this purpose owing to the strong symbolic value of food and its ability to saturate all areas of human pleasure. The finding of feeding methods that are as safe as possible falls, in our opinion, among the skills of the staff involved in palliative medicine and justifies the presence of the deglutologist speech therapist in this particular area of health care.

Chapter 1 addresses the various meanings of the meal. In fact, the meal, increasingly referred to by the English term *mealtime*, has taken on different forms and methods of implementation over different periods, and today, it has different characteristics in different geographical areas. The meal, in all cultures and at all latitudes, albeit with inevitable exceptions, is an expression of conviviality that is expressed in the observance of certain procedural and aesthetic rules. These take the form of real ceremonies on the occasion of official lunches and special occasions that mark the life of a community or of an individual. The meal is consumed at specific times, which, like all aspects of human life, have been subject to variations and modifications over time, adapting to the transformations of social living. Moreover, food and meals take on a special meaning in religious life, particularly in monastic life, where faith is lived in a community dimension.

Chapter 2 analyzes the meaning of dysphagia by illustrating its spread through the analysis of incidence and prevalence rates of different diseases. Dysphagia leads to the onset of different consequences for the health status of dysphagic individuals. Malnutrition and dehydration are among the most relevant aspects because of the serious consequences they have on the nutritional status of the subject. The relationship between malnutrition and dysphagia is somewhat circular; in fact, dysphagia causes malnutrition, but in turn, malnutrition causes dysphagia. It therefore becomes important to break as soon as possible a vicious cycle that inevitably leads patients to serious and extreme consequences. Dysphagia increases the likelihood, already present in all subjects who eat, that food may accidentally end up in the airways. The popular saying "When you eat you fight with death," despite the terrible scenarios it depicts, is not without foundation. The accidental introduction of food into airways can block them, thus preventing the passage of air, or can cause inflammatory phenomena when smaller boluses contaminated by bacteria reach the lung cavities. Finally, difficulty swallowing often leads to isolation and social withdrawal due to the discomfort of participating in the ritual of a common meal. This factor determines the worsening of the subject's quality of life, and in some cases, it persists even in subjects who have successfully followed a rehabilitative path. In fact, the adoption of particular strategies to make meals safe for dysphagic individuals can often favor their distance from common meals. Therefore, professionals who deal with dysphagia must take care not only of the safety and restoration of swallowing functionality but also of reintegrating the subject into the normal eating routine.

Chapter 3 analyzes the assessment of dysphagia. The detection of and knowledge of swallowing problems are prejudicial for the adoption of any remedial strategy. To date, despite the availability of a number of swallowing difficulty assessment tools for clinicians, their use is not widespread. Such an attitude exposes patients, especially those advanced in age, to serious risks of developing the consequences that, as seen in Chap. 2, characterize the presence of dysphagia. The culture of assessing swallowing disorders must spread as quickly as possible among healthcare professionals, who, each for their specific professional competence, are called to assist patients potentially exposed to dysphagia. The evaluation of dysphagia is divided into three different levels, each of which, with specific techniques, involves health professionals. Particular concern is due to *meal observation,* an evaluative method that examines the entire duration of the meal, during which qualitative phenomena may occur, possibly undetected in the previous three-levels of evaluation.

Chapter 4 analyzes all the intervention tools available to the speech therapist for the treatment of patients with dysphagia. Deglutology is a relatively young discipline; however, in its short history, it has accumulated a considerable amount of knowledge on the act of swallowing and on the possibility of effectively intervening in its dysfunctions. As often occurs in clinical practice, the urgency of providing answers in the field of assistance has preceded research on the validity of the proposed intervention tools. The same happens in the field of deglutology, where many of the techniques commonly used are still waiting for necessary efficacy studies. In recent years, considerable effort has been made to provide the necessary scientific support to many established practices and to equip clinicians with new intervention methods. Many of these new methods are still experimental, but it is hoped that they can soon become clinical tools of common use. Currently, three types of approaches can be applied to patients with dysphagia. The first, the *compensatory approach*, consists of the search for strategies that ensure the restoration of swallowing functionality, even in the presence of symptoms causing dysphagia. This mode of intervention constitutes the historical core of dysphagia management, and it still retains its validity, for which it is massively employed by speech therapists. The *rehabilitative approach*, owing to cues from recent theories, primarily new statements on neuroplasticity, has undergone significant acceleration in recent years. Many exercises and intervention protocols for specific swallowing difficulties are now available to rehabilitators. Finally, *preventive strategies* aim to prevent or minimize the effects of dysphagia in patients undergoing chemoradiotherapy for head–neck district neoplasms. A strong interest in this type of approach has been developing since the 2000s, with a significant increase in the last 6 years.

Chapter 5 explores the close link between quality of life and nutrition and analyzes in detail the methods required to ensure the maximum safety of a person with dysphagia at a meal. In fact, subjects with medium or mild dysphagia, although they frequently have limitations, can continue to consume food during meals. However, this must occur according to some fundamental rules that normally have universal validity but that take on a prescriptive meaning in patients with dysphagia. Indeed, the meal of a person with dysphagia must take place while respecting certain postural conditions and in environmental contexts provided with particular features. Moreover, food must faithfully meet the characteristics expressed in the evaluation of patients with dysphagia. It is also good practice for those who assist in the meals of children, even nondysphagic ones, and people with dysphagia to be able to implement the most common antichoking techniques. The care of oral hygiene and health has a meaning, not only in social life but also in the prevention of lung inflammation phenomena. Research in recent years has highlighted the close link between oral hygiene and the onset of aspiration pneumonia. Oral hygiene is, therefore, a fundamental aspect in the management of patients with dysphagia, which does not lose its meaning even in subjects who no longer eat by mouth. In these patients, the aspiration of saliva can still cause the transfer of bacterial agents from the mouth to the lungs, with the consequent risk of the onset of inflammatory phenomena.

This chapter concludes with an exploration of the concept of *palliative feeding*, namely feeding that no longer has a nutritional meaning but is carried out for the sole purpose of positively impacting the quality of life of the individual. In this sense, the presence of a speech therapist becomes significant within the team that takes care of patients in the last stage of their life. When the meal, despite the restrictions imposed by the disease, is exclusively practiced for hedonistic purposes, it is essential for the patient to express their own desires and tastes to avoid the imposition of unwanted choices. It is therefore necessary to know and manage the tools of augmentative alternative communication (AAC) that can help the clinician and the caregiver collect requests from the sick person and then satisfy them.

A book is born in the present, but it is a child of our history, and in some way, it testifies to the desire to leave a trace in the future. I am pleased, as well as obliged, to thank those who have contributed to enabling me to write this text. Thanking them all one by one would require such a long list that it would probably induce the reader to skip it wholly. However, I cannot fail to thank Professor Oskar Schindler, the undisputed master of Italian deglutology, to whom all deglutologists owe a tribute of recognition. I have an additional debt with Oskar, who was able to stand by me in some challenging moments of my life. The preface of this book should have been by Professor Oskar Schindler. Unfortunately, fate did not give us the time. I hope that Oskar can appreciate this work from the dimension of light in which he surely finds himself now: "Dear Oskar, our project is only postponed to another dimension." I thank Giovanni Ruoppolo, a professor at Sapienza University of Rome, and a lifelong friend. I thank Carmelina Razzano, my teacher, to whom I owe the rigor with which I faced the speech therapy profession. Jokingly, but not quite, I have always called Carmelina "my super speech therapy ego" and now, on in years and in my career, I just can reiterate this youthful definition. Thanks to Chiara and my family: they supported or better tolerated me during the long gestation and preparation of this volume. I would like to thank Floriana and Mauro, who reviewed the linguistic stumbles of the text. A special thanks goes to the travel companions who shared with me the effort of writing some chapters of this book, as well as to Giulia, Marianna, and Nicoletta, who took on the burden of reading the chapters and giving me valuable suggestions. I thank Antonella, my editor, for her advice and for encouraging me to persist in the enterprise during these difficult times.

Thank you to my students, whose doubts urged me to further investigate and better clarify some basic concepts of deglutology. I thank the many patients who over the years have driven me to constantly expand and deepen my knowledge, never considering myself satisfied, always in search of new solutions to swallowing problems. Lastly, a thank you to the readers, hopefully not a few of them, who both for the joy of the publisher and mine (why not?) will have the initiative to buy this book and even more to read it. To this book, I wish a destiny not as a decorative complement but as a useful tool for those who strive for the well-being of people with dysphagia daily.

Disclaimer The translation of passages quoted from texts without an Italian edition was made by the author. The last access to the Internet pages indicated in the volume was made in June 2021.

Contents

1 The Human at the Table 1
1.1 The Meal as Conviviality 2
1.2 The Aesthetics of the Meal 5
1.3 Mealtimes 8
1.4 The Meal in Monastic Life 9
References 11

2 Dysphagia in Adulthood and the Geriatric Age 13
2.1 Incidence and Prevalence of Dysphagia 16
2.2 The Consequences of Dysphagia 19
2.2.1 Malnutrition 20
2.2.2 The Passage of a Food Bolus into the Airways 21
2.2.3 The Psychosocial Consequences 24
2.3 Clinical Management of Dysphagic Patients 24
2.3.1 Professionals Involved in the Management of Patients with Dysphagia 25
2.3.2 Different Care Settings for Dysphagic Patients 27
2.4 Speech Therapy Management of Patients with Dysphagia 28
References 29

3 Assessment of Dysphagia in Adult Dysphagic Patients 35
3.1 Clinical Evaluation 37
3.1.1 Dysphagia Screening 38
3.1.2 Clinical Swallow Examination 44
3.2 Instrumental Evaluation 49
3.3 Mealtime Observation 50
References 54

4 Treatment of Dysphagia in Adult Dysphagic Patients 57
4.1 Compensation Strategies 58
4.1.1 Postural Compensation 58
4.1.2 Dietary Compensation 62
4.2 Rehabilitative Strategies 70
4.2.1 Principles of Exercise: Neuroplasticity 71
4.2.2 *Isometric Progressive Resistance Oropharyngeal* (I-PRO) *Therapy*: Isometric Tongue Exercises 73

4.2.3 Rehabilitation Protocols 78
4.2.4 Functional Stimulation (Skill-Based Rehabilitation) 79
4.2.5 Biofeedback 81
4.2.6 Indirect Electrical Stimulation 81
4.3 Maneuvers 84
4.3.1 The Forced Swallowing Maneuver 85
4.3.2 Decomposition of Swallowing 85
4.3.3 Supraglottic and Super-supraglottic Swallowing Maneuvers 86
4.3.4 Multiple Swallows 87
4.3.5 Shaker Maneuver 88
4.3.6 Masako Maneuver 88
4.3.7 Mendelsohn Maneuver 89
4.3.8 Rapid Mandibular Opening Maneuver 90
4.4 Preventive Strategies 90
References 92

5 The Meal of the Person with Dysphagia 101
5.1 Quality of Life and Nutrition 101
5.2 The Meal Setting 105
5.2.1 Posture 106
5.2.2 The Characteristics of Food 109
5.2.3 The Characteristics of the Setting and the Behavior of the Caregiver 111
5.2.4 Emergency Management 114
5.2.5 Oral Hygiene 115
5.3 Palliative Feeding 118
5.3.1 Speech Therapy Assistance for Oncological Patients in Palliative Care 119
5.3.2 Communicating Food Choices 124
5.3.3 *Low-Technology Aids* (Low-Tech) 132
5.3.4 The Communicative Partners 135
References 136

Appendix 141

1 The Human at the Table

Humans spend part of their day at the table where they consume their meals. The term "meal" can be replaced with *mealtime* which similarly, in English, indicates the time that, in different ways and forms, is dedicated to eating. When we talk about eating, we often indifferently use the terms "feeding" or "nutrition" even though, in reality, they express different concepts. In fact, "feeding" refers to the intake of an organism of the foods essential to its metabolism and its daily vital functions; "nutrition," on the other hand, refers to the set of biological processes that allow humans to absorb and use all the food substances ingested, which are necessary for the survival of the organism. Feeding is strongly influenced by cultural aspects, whereas nutrition is based on biological processes. *How* and *what* we eat are linked to the geographical and cultural context in which we feed; what we eat is also linked to the absorption capacity of the human digestive system, for which some foods are edible and others are not. This means that nutrition is connected to the evolution of the species; for example, in the case of humans, the digestive system is unsuitable for absorbing woody substances (Consiglio and Siani 2003; Lévi-Strauss 2016). What we eat does not depend only on biological aspects but is also strongly connected to cultural aspects such as the consumption of the meat of some animals, which is allowed in certain cultural contexts and forbidden or considered taboo in others. Pork meat has a different treatment in the three great Western monotheistic religions: Christian religion allows its consumption, which is instead forbidden by the Jewish and Muslim religions. An example of food taboo is dog meat, which is regularly consumed in Southeast Asia but is a taboo for the Western world, where this animal is considered a *pet*. In the Anglo-Saxon world, horse meat is considered taboo which, on the contrary, is normally consumed in the rest of Europe. For all cultures the absolute taboo is the consumption of human meat. Eating is often the beginning and cement of friendly and affectionate relationships in general. How many affectionate relationships start with a coffee and are cemented in dinners among friends! The working breakfast testifies to the importance of the convivial moment in working life, when professional speech takes on an apparently

A. Amitrano, *Dysphagia and Nutrition*,
https://doi.org/10.1007/978-3-031-77449-2_1

hedonistic guise, but, in reality, essential to advance important professional relationships. It can be fully stated that food and the act of eating are elements that pervade different aspects of our life and go beyond the strictly nutritional meaning (Fischler 1992). The role that eating has in quality of life is widely recognized and confirmed by common sense. The survey carried out during the Expo of Milan in 2015 indicated the preferences of the sample which consisted of more than a thousand families interviewed on the sidelines of the trade fair event: for most of the sample, eating is one of the greatest pleasures of life, 8% eat only to live, and another 8% considers eating as the main pleasure of life. Literature as well variously reiterates this concept: "Eating is one of the four purposes of life... what the other three are, no one has ever known" (Chinese proverb), "One cannot think well, love well, sleep well, if one has not eaten well" (Virginia Woolf), "Meditate well on this point: the best hours of our life are all connected, with a more or less tangible link, to some memory of the table" (Charles Pierre Monselet), "Man is what he eats" (Ludwig Feuerbach), and "The best things in life are either immoral, or are illegal, or make you gain weight" (George Bernard Shaw).

1.1 The Meal as Conviviality

Food is an element of cultural identity that richly represents the history, evolution, and religion of people (Amitrano and Bonazzi 2011; Amitrano and Ruoppolo 2014). At the same time, food is "the most accessible threshold of a culture," and "eating the cuisine of others means crossing this threshold" (Montanari 2002, 2004, 2009). Food somehow expresses itself—"Tell me what you eat and I will tell you who you are" (Brillat-Savarin 2002)—and is commonly assumed during the *meal* which defines the time when food is consumed. Meals have their own subdivision throughout the day, which inevitably ends up marking the rhythm and cyclicity. In our culture, breakfast precedes lunch, which, in turn, as the day progresses, is consumed before dinner. Each meal has its own characterization derived from the geographical and cultural context, as well as individual preferences. Breakfast, for example, is, for some, simply coffee; for others, it is richer in food, generally sweet and almost never salty or fried, which in contrast constitutes the main element of breakfast in the Anglo-Saxon world. Regardless of the time of day and the richness or lack of the menu, the meal is an occasion for social participation. Even in a professional context, breakfast and business lunch are important relational moments for establishing alliances and concluding deals. In fact humans love to eat in groups, unlike other living beings, who feed in solitude, who are careful to defend their food from thieves and predators. Plutarch has one of the characteristics of *convivial disputes*: "We do not invite each other to eat and drink simply, but to eat and drink together." Cicero claimed that, "the pleasure of banquets should not be measured by the delicacy of the dishes, but by the company of friends and their conversations." Even in modern times, sharing remains an essential element of nutrition: conviviality is a characteristic element of human rationality, a crucial moment of exchange and intimate relationships with those close to us (Meglio 2012).

In the Middle Ages, whoever shares bread with someone becomes his "companion." The term derives from the vernacular *companion*, which is composed of cum/*com* ("together, with") and *panis* ("bread") and is literally "bread companion." Even the word *convivio*, a refined definition of the meal, has its root in cum-*vivere*, that is, "living together"—a living together to which the sharing of the meal that unites all social classes gives sense, value, and meaning. Even the peasant family in the Middle Ages defines its identity at the table: "Living on one bread and one wine," or sharing the same meal, was and remains a way to indicate belonging to the same family group.

Participation in a common meal is, in different cultures, the first sign of belonging to the group. On Tonga Islands, in the Pacific, if a man and a woman eat together a particular food, they are engaged; if they eat another, they are automatically married. The participation in the common meal is the identity root not only of the family group but also of larger communities: every association or brotherhood has in conviviality a moment of strengthening the group spirit. In monastic communities, the confreres consume together the meal in the silence of the refectory, listening to the word of the Lord and nourishing at the same time the body and the spirit. Conviviality is the essence of some dishes and the ways in which they are consumed. In Piedmont, the *bagna càuda* is brought to the table in a single container, the *diàn or fojot,* from which everyone draws. Even the French *bourguignonne*, the Swiss *fondue*, the Maghreb *cous cous*, and the Ethiopian *zighinì* involve similar rituals. The rule of sharing does not exclude exceptions: for example, the famous Commissioner Montalbano, in *The Terracotta Dog*, "Took the dishes, a bottle of wine, the bread, turns on the television, sits down at the table. He liked to eat alone, to enjoy bites in silence." The commissioner has nothing to rebut to his deputy, Augello, who, in Montalbano's arancini, tells him, "The real truth is that you like to eat alone," because his thought on the matter is that, "Tasting a dish made as God commands is one of the most refined pleasures that man can enjoy, not to be shared with anyone, not even with the person you love the most." Eating alone generally has a negative connotation, and in some traditions, it is almost a taboo, as evidenced by the following proverbs: "who eats alone chokes in solitude" (Arab proverb), "He who eats alone chokes" (Roman proverb), "Anyone who eats alone chokes" (Ciociaro proverb), "If you eat alone you choke" (Salento proverb), and "who does not drink in company is either a thief or a spy" (proverb of popular tradition). The web society is bringing noticeable changes to the sociability of eating; in fact, it is not uncommon to see diners absorbed in consulting their own device. Diners have their meals accompanied by their tablet or smartphone, in connection with others, thus creating a new kind of commensality: the virtual one, which brings us closer to those who are far away, effectively distancing us from those who are close. The meal, in its community dimension, does not necessarily mean peaceful and equal relationships among the diners. In fact, if the common meal testifies to belonging to the social group, it is also true that it represents its stratifications. Hierarchical roles are indeed well represented in the arrangement around the table, where the place is not assigned at random; in a more or less formalized way at different ages, it signals the importance and prestige of the diners: the leader in the center and the others at a distance inversely proportional to the role that is recognized to each. Depending on the times and social and political contexts, the arrangement at the table serves to indicate the leader and the hierarchical positions within the group. At the court of Byzantium, in the tenth century, Liutprand, bishop of Cremona and ambassador of Otto I of Saxony, was placed at the table in the 15th position, at a distance from the sovereign that the interested party did not consider suitable for his role, and this did not fail to create a serious diplomatic incident. Even Dante happens, tells Giovanni Sercambi in one of his novellas, to be placed in a peripheral position at a banquet at the court of Naples. Since the king wanted the supreme poet as a guest "In order to see and hear of his wisdom and virtue," he invited him to his court. But when he arrived "dressed quite cheaply, as poets usually used," he was not identified, and at lunchtime, "water was given to the hands and they went to the table, the king at his table and the other barons seated; finally, Dante was put at the end of the table." Offended by the treatment reserved for him, "he ate and immediately left […] to go back to Tuscany." Realizing the misunderstanding, the king had him chased by a servant with a letter of apology. The poet, once reached by the servant and having accepted the king's apologies, returned to Naples, but this time, "he dressed in a very beautiful robe." At the next banquet, the poet was seated at the king's side, but during the meal, he behaved quite bizarrely: "taking the meat, and on the chest and up on the clothes, he rubbed it; so the wine he rubbed on the clothes." When the king asked for an explanation of such bizarreness, he replied: "Holy crown, I recognize that this great honor that is now done, you have done to the clothes; and therefore I wanted the clothes to enjoy the prepared food." The king, recognizing the honesty and wisdom of the poet, "made him stay in court to be able to hear more" (Sercambi 1974, *passim*).

The hierarchical representation in the table arrangement reaches its peak in absolute monarchy, where the king does not share the table with anyone, thus representing his otherness from the rest of the courtiers. In patriarchal contexts, the head of the family always sits at the head of the table, the short side of the rectangle that draws the table, which is generally set for only one diner. From this perspective, the round table expresses a characteristic of democracy in its poor ability to signal differences and hierarchies. In fact, the famous round table of King Arthur was the symbol of the absolute equality of those who were part of it. Moreover, the presence at the table indicates being there, and the fact of continuing to set for who is gone must be interpreted in this sense. Moreover, around the table, it is preferable to sit only a certain number of diners, never 13 or 17. In these cases, to neutralize the ominous omens, it is traditional to set for a 14th nonexistent guest, whose food is then evenly divided among the 13 present. This is a very ancient superstition that dates back to the Last Supper, in which the presence of 13 diners preceded the death of Jesus. A pre-Christian matrix can be found in Scandinavian mythology that tells of a feast of 12 gods, to which Loki, the deity of conflict and evil, tries to join, increasing the number of diners to 13. The events that followed the unwanted intrusion led to the death of Balder, the favorite of the gods. The pleasure of the table can be achieved whenever four conditions are met: tasty meat, good wine, amiable guests, and sufficient time (Brillat-Savarin 2002).

1.2 The Aesthetics of the Meal

The meal expresses our aesthetic taste in different ways, including the setting of the table, which, while responding to very precise rules codified in a specific etiquette ad hoc, manifests the taste and wealth, not only artistic, of those who set. The care of the table plays an important role in personal and collective situations. Think, for example, of the Christmas table or the birthday party table. According to Lanza (2016), the table, a highly ritualized daily practice, is considered a metaphor for life. In a relatively small stage, i.e., elbow to elbow, a representation that reproduces different aspects of reality takes place. One of the first testimonies on the history of the table is the curse launched by the queen of the Harpies, Celeno, in the third song of the *Aeneid*, to Aeneas and his warriors, to whom she wished "so much hunger that you will even bite the tables." In reality, Aeneas and his brave warriors had to eat the *mensae*, that is, those discs of bread that the maids distributed at the beginning of lunch and that served as plates on which the foods were placed and therefore collected the juices and leftovers of the food. At the end of lunch, the *mensae* were given to beggars. For the warriors, eating the mensae was a degrading act but was certainly not contrary to the rules of the human digestive system. The oldest pizzas in history, soaked in the juices and remains of the foods that had been placed on them to be cut, were eaten by the companions of the son of Venus (Rebora 1998). The *mensae*, which generally served two diners, were gradually replaced by a cutting board, a wooden or ceramic dish, which was already present in Italy in the twelfth century. In the fifteenth century, in Italy before elsewhere, the use of plates, as well as individual glass and forks, spread. The fork arrived in Italy with the dowry of the Byzantine princess Theodora Ducasche, who married Doge Domenico Selvo in 1071. The "pironia" (from the Greek *peìrein*, "to pierce"), a two-pronged gold fork introduced at court by the young bride, caused quite a stir. In Florence, the Medici banned its use, considering it indecent. The Church, for its part, called the fork a diabolical tool. Before reaching its current use, two- or three-pronged forks, forged in precious metals and adorned with equally precious stones, were exclusively for fruit. The first fork given to a king on record is the one given in 1380 to Charles V, the king of France. In the nineteenth century, a special fork was created, *à melon*, flat and with very short prongs, which was used to eat melon. The flat part was used to cut the melon into pieces, and the small prongs were used to bring them to the mouth. The knife has a more ancient presence on the table and was in fact the only cutlery in use in the Middle Ages, when it was used both to cut meat and to bring it to the mouth. It was not uncommon to use it as a substitute for a toothpick (Lévi-Strauss 1999). Glasses, the fruit of the ingenuity of glass masters, gradually replaced the precious metal cups that were part of the individual trousseau of every nobleman. Glasses slowly diversify, taking on a specific shape depending on the type of liquid they are intended to contain (Standage 2005). The proliferation of dishes of different shapes and uses made it very complicated to set the table, a task reserved for the servants who, coming from the less affluent classes, were not used to the variety of dishes and dishes. It was therefore necessary to create specific manuals to help the perfect housewife instruct the service staff. In establishing the rules for setting the table, a significant place must be given to Monsignor della Casa, who, in *Galateo*, dictated the rules of civil living. The setting of the table thus becomes a theory that finds functionality as its founding criterion. In fact, the place that the cutlery occupies in relation to the plate depends on its use during the meal. The fork goes on the left because it is with the left hand that it is held to facilitate the sectioning of the dish with the knife, held with the right hand. The knife and the spoon, indeed, go strictly to the right; the former is closer to the plate and the latter is more external. Both cutleries are therefore used by the right hand, and generally, the spoon, which is useful for removing broths and soups, is used before the knife. This is no longer pointed like the medieval cutlery but almost always has a rounded tip, initially adopted to discourage its use as a toothpick and, later, to temper its vaguely threatening appearance. The presence of the napkin has a long history: the ancient Romans tied a *mantelium*, usually made of linen, around their necks to clean their hands and protect their tunic during meals consumed on the triclinium. Under the toga, however, the *mappa*, which was used at the end of the meal to collect left-over food and take it home, was hidden. In the Middle Ages, the *touaille* was used to clean hands during the banquet and was placed on the table or, sometimes, hung on a wall, such as a curtain. In the late Middle Ages, a napkin for cleaning hands was distinct from the one for wiping lips before drinking. In the seventeenth century, the napkin also underwent the influence of Baroque, and, scented with delicate essences, it was present on the tables with refined pleats that give it zoomorphic or mythological shapes. The napkin is no longer used only for the cleanliness of the diner but also to cover the bread or the plate while waiting for the start of lunch. Over the centuries, the napkin followed a "descending" path: initially, it was placed on the shoulder; then, progressively, it moved to the forearm (as was used in the seventeenth century and as old-style waiters still do), until it reached the thigh as we all used it (Lanza 2016). In the etiquette of table setting, the napkin must be strictly on the left and never under the cutlery, to allow the diner to unfold it with two fingers and place it on the legs. An element that embellishes the meal table is the centerpiece, a composition generally floral, which aims to enhance the table and underline the importance of the event to be celebrated. The centerpiece did not always play an exclusively aesthetic role. Initially, it was an expression of the importance of the banquet organizer; it bore the family crest and reflected the family's wealth through the materials with which it was made. Later, ceramics and majolica replaced the centerpieces of metals and precious stones, but with their splendor, they did not stop representing the power and wealth of the banquet organizer. Over the centuries, the centerpiece has stripped itself of this need and has increasingly taken on a value exclusively aesthetic. Floral elements and original details have gradually replaced valuable materials, making the centerpiece an ephemeral element and unsuitable for conservation. The aesthetics of the table are fundamental and not secondary to the care that is dedicated to oneself. It is important to prepare an adequate setup even when one has lunch alone. "Lucullus dines with Lucullus" is the reproach that Lucullus made to the servant, who, since the master was dining alone, had prepared the table in a less sumptuous way than what he did on the occasion of the usual banquets with friends. The reproach implies that all the attention that the host required for himself or herself was no less than for his or her guests.

The aesthetics of food do not end in the aesthetics of the table but are somehow inherent in the food itself, whose presentation is intimately connected to the notion of appetibility, that is, the ability of foods to make themselves desirable before being tasted (Marchesi and Vercelloni 2001). Mouthwatering, a typical sensation associated with good food, is aroused by organoleptic parameters of food, such as aroma, shape, color, and the environment. All these dimensions significantly affect the level of food liking. In the 1930s, the English food scientist Moir (1936) organized for his colleagues the "banquet of chromatic counterfeits": a meal based on dishes prepared with top-quality ingredients and impeccably cooked but artificially colored in an unusual way. Numerous banquet participants reported nausea and discomfort because the colors ordinarily associated with food were out of place. Moir also reported that, in the presence of chromatic distortions, the recognition of fruit jellies occurred erroneously. On the basis of these experiences, English food scientists deduced the role of the bewitching faculty of color in the recognition of food. Other experiments have further documented the difficulties encountered by the taster in recognizing a syrup colored in an atypical way. Additionally, in the field of wine, it is known how much the visual impact of wine is reflected in the tasting process. The expert taster entrusts to the chromatic characteristics of precise qualitative indications: it is said that the color is a bit like the appearance of the wine: its age and the character (Peynaud 1980). Wine tasting is significantly misled by visual disturbances, consisting of colored glasses and dim or deceptive lights. Drinking blindfolded, it is easy to confuse a white low in acidity with a red full of tannins. During an experiment, a group of graduates from the Faculty of Enology in Bordeaux (Morrot et al. 2001) were invited to taste red wine and white wine. The expert tasters described the typical characteristics of a red wine as a white wine, unknowingly colored red. Sight, therefore, makes taste abilities more efficient or, in some cases, can mislead them. This fact has important commercial implications: an orange juice with a deep orange color is generally considered better than a pale yellow juice. Attention to color also extends to food packaging, which acts not only as an incentive to purchase but also as a psychological integration to taste. An unfortunate coloring produces inhibitory effects on the consumer. In sugar packages, care is taken to avoid greening, which is generally associated with astringency; in contrast, blue, the color of sweetness, is preferred. Information, however, can change our attitude toward colors. This is evidence of the recent aversion to artificial colors, which are often used in the production of brightly colored drinks. Today, once the harmfulness of most dyes has been proven, drinks are put on the market in a faded version that, not long ago, would not have aroused the slightest attraction in potential consumers.

Goethe was among the first to notice the influence of individual colors on the onset of specific moods. Observing a landscape through yellow glass stimulates serenity and cheerfulness (Goethe 1999). Red color gives rise to states of excitement, whereas blue gives sensations of tenderness, restlessness, and nostalgia. Subsequent experimental research has documented the substantial truth of the poet's conclusions. The associations of colors with psychological states have been variously interpreted. Luscher (1976) traces them back to man's ancestral experiences: light colors, such as yellow, are linked to daytime experiences and therefore to activity, whereas colors close to blue evoke the night and therefore the slowing down of vital activities. Specifically, the colors of food often determine our disposition toward consumption. On the basis of experience and education, food is assigned a stereotyped image judged as indicative of nutritional properties and edibility, as well as the state of ripeness or preservation. Many of the clues detected are found, such as green indicating bitterness or red and yellow testifying to the occurrence of ripening or traces of mold that, with the bluish coloration, indicate the beginning of the putrefaction of the food in question. Similarly, the regularity of shape, the uniformity of color, and the appearance of the surface are visual qualities that are associated with food hygiene. However, irrational prejudices are often held, such as considering brightly colored egg yolk more nutritious or greenish-colored oil more genuine. The aesthetic characteristics of food itself are further enhanced by plating. The arrangement of food on serving dishes plays an important role in the success of a dish. A carefully presented dish has a strong psychological impact on the taster who, also from aesthetics, will derive his disposition to tasting. As a famous chef says, the composition of the dish is much more than an aesthetic fact: it is form, substance, and meaning—because a plating works when it reflects a preparation process (Cracco 2015). The beauty of a table and food is not just an aesthetic experience but is also closely related to taste and therefore to the pleasure we derive from the food itself. The shape of the food, its placement on the plate, and its visual characteristics all enhance the taste, preceding the encounter through smell and sight. As sometimes happens with all human things, even the aesthetic search for food can be exacerbated in extreme forms. Today, it is quite common to see people at the table photographing food to share images immediately on social media. The term *food photography* is a very widespread activity. On the web, platforms such as Chewsy, Evernote Food, and Foodspotting are dedicated to photos of users who share images of their own food. The term *food porn*, which first appeared in 1984, indicates a phenomenon that has become increasingly widespread and describes a tendency to create and share images of food that stimulate excitement and an impulse to eat it. The food thus represented is lustful, sensual, but not low quality or to be ingested quickly and caloric, but it is beautiful to look at and to share (Cucciniello 2010).

1.3 Mealtimes

Meals take place at predetermined times and follow a rhythm that seems natural to us until we encounter the rhythms used in other geographical areas, where our established habits are completely overturned by different rhythms and times. Long trips around the world are not necessary to observe such changes; just across the regions of Italy, one can witness often the irrelevant changes in the amount of time when daily meals are consumed. Additionally, the times when the meal is served vary depending on the situations in which it is consumed. Consider, for example, the times when dinner is served in hospitals. The distribution of meals during the day and the way they are consumed significantly differ across geographical regions and cultures. This aspect is also subject to the effects of globalization, which tends to standardize the times and ways of the meal; an example is the spread of McDonald's restaurants worldwide. The rhythm of meals marks the flow of the day and plays a secondary role in temporal orientation. Even the rhythm of meals, such as their hourly placement and composition, follows sociological factors with their own history, which has marked significant changes over the centuries. Mealtimes, in fact, are a cultural construction and therefore differ from one country to another, from one social class to another, and from one era to another. At the beginning of the eighteenth century, the meals of the rich began with a breakfast that, in the international lexicon of the wealthy classes, was called *déjeuner*; followed by a hearty lunch, the *diner*, consumed between one and two o'clock; and finally a light dinner, the *souper*, consumed in the evening. Between the end of the eighteenth century and the beginning of the nineteenth century in European aristocracy, starting with the English one, there was a progressive temporal shift of the main meal, that is, the French *diner*, the English *dinner*, and the Italian *pranzo* (*lunch*), which slowly moved toward the late hours of the afternoon. In fact, the wealthy classes, who stayed late in the evening, engaged in dances and shows, got up just as late in the morning and consequently had breakfast at a time very close to that of lunch. The traditional midday meal thus moved toward the late afternoon, at five or six, almost overlapping with dinner, which, in fact, was replaced by a light meal consumed late at night, after the shows. Eating late became a real *status symbol* of the wealthy social class, as reported in numerous literary quotations. The progressive shift ended at the end of the first war. This shift has left a trace in the lexicon, and in fact, in Paris, *déjeuner* is the midday meal, and *diner* is dinner. The same is true in English, where *dinner* no longer indicates the midday meal, today *lunch*, but the evening meal.

1.4 The Meal in Monastic Life

Monasteries are considered, not wrongly, places of great gastronomic culture. There are several recipe books that come from the kitchens of monasteries and that pass on to the world the elements of a cuisine made of simple and genuine ingredients. The *Dictionnaire de gastronomie* reports that "towards the end of the Merovingian age, the convents, holders of all gastronomic traditions, multiplied in France, thus giving a great impulse to culinary art." However, how did the monks consume their meals? Precise indications come from the rule of St. Benedict, which, although written fifteen centuries ago, has still been successfully applied on five continents (AA.VV 2016). The rule describes not only the foods and their quantities that the monks must consume in the various seasons of the year but also the ways in which the meal must be consumed. Monks eat at the same time: "No one is allowed to eat or drink anything before the established time." Needless to emphasize the value of this rule strengthens the sense of community. Monks eat at the same table, serving each other. In the refectory where a monk, during meals, reads passages from the Bible or the life of a saint, silence reigns: "In the refectory there should be a deep silence, so that no whisper or voice is heard, except that of the reader." The monks' table is not at all poor: "Two cooked dishes should be sufficient; if there is the possibility of getting fresh fruit or vegetables, add a third. For bread, I think a generous kilo per day is enough, whether there is only one meal or when there is lunch and dinner. If the daily work has been heavier than usual, if the Abbot deems it appropriate, he will have full power to add a small supplement," but it is added, "provided that all abuse is absolutely avoided and the monk guards against greed, because nothing is so unbecoming for a Christian, as the excesses of the table." When the monk's work is more strenuous, the rule provides for the possibility of more abundant meals. You can drink at the table, but moderately: "Taking into account the frail constitution of the most delicate, we believe that a quarter of wine per head can suffice for everyone," because "wine makes the wise apostate." Additionally, for wine, an exception is provided under special conditions: "If, however, the local needs or work or the summer heat required a greater quantity, it is in the power of the superior to grant it, always taking care to avoid satiety and even more drunkness." Abstinence from wine remains a positive value: "As for the brothers who have received from God the strength to abstain from it completely, know that they will receive a special reward."

The meal of Carthusian monks is solitary and finds its community dimension only on Sunday, when it is consumed in the common refectory (Peters 2011). At 12:00, the Angelus rings, and while the monks direct their prayer to Mary, a lay brother or an employee of the Charterhouse puts lunch in the food pass that is next to the door of the cell, overlooking the cloister. The food pass has two doors that, with respect to the intimacy and solitude of the cell, are never opened at the same time. After the sixth hour, the monk arranges the food left on the food pass in the refectory of the cell, and a table is arranged near the window that, in special drawers, keeps the necessary to consume the meal: cutlery, napkin, salt, oil, vinegar, and water. The consumption of a meal usually takes place in solitude after the recitation of a prayer. The participants were not allowed to study during lunch. The monks, except for certain times of the year, consume only one meal of simple and tasty foods. The dishes are hot and accompanied by salad and cheese. Meat does not enter the menu on any occasion. On Fridays or the eve of solemnities, the monks are content to eat bread and drink water. Special attention is finally given to the refectory in the convents, the room where, in all buildings intended for collective living, the meal is generally consumed.

The refectory was important and predominant in ancient monastic constructions, where it often constituted the only place for collective gathering. In fact, while in more modern convents, and in those in the West, there were various rooms intended for gathering or for common work such as chapter halls, libraries, workshops, warehouses, etc., in the oldest eastern monasteries, the refectory was the only large room where the monks gathered. The refectories of the Greek Orthodox convents consist of a rectangular room, which is very elongated in shape and is mostly covered by a barrel vault. On one of the short sides, there is a small apse, which is the place of the *hegoùmenos*, the superior, who sits at the end of a long and narrow table, often made of stone, that runs the entire length of the refectory. The table of the Néa Monḗ convent, on the island of Chios, dating back to the eleventh century, has a top with a geometric inlay, whereas the massive sides contain many tiny niches where each diner could store their modest table service.

References

AA.VV. La regola di San Benedetto. Camerata Picena: Shalom Editrice; 2016.
Amitrano A, Bonazzi C. Alimentazione e disfagia: aspetti interculturali. In: Schindler O, Ruoppolo G, Schindler A, editors. Deglutologia. Torino: Omega Edizioni; 2011.
Amitrano A., Ruoppolo G. (2014), L'alimentazione nelle diverse culture, in D. Patrocinio, A. Schindler I disturbi della comunicazione nella popolazione multiculturale e multilingue, FrancoAngeli, Milano.
Brillat-Savarin JA. Fisiologia del gusto. Torino: Edizioni SEB27; 2002.
Consiglio C, Siani V. Evoluzione e alimentazione. Torino: Bollati Boringhieri; 2003.
Cracco C. In principio era l'anguria salata. Viaggio al centro del gusto. Milano: Rizzoli; 2015.
Cucciniello C. Food porn, la seduzione del cibo, L'Espresso Food and Wine, 21 settembre 2010.
Fischler C. L'onnivoro. Il piacere di mangiare nella storia e nella scienza. Milano: Mondadori; 1992.
Goethe JW. La teoria dei colori. Milano: il Saggiatore; 1999.
Lanza E. Il tovagliolo va a sinistra. Milano: Vallardi; 2016.
Lévi-Strauss C. Le origini delle buone maniere a tavola. Milano: il Saggiatore; 1999.
Lévi-Strauss C. Il crudo e il cotto. Milano: il Saggiatore; 2016.
Luscher M. Il test dei colori. Roma: Astrolabio; 1976.
Marchesi G, Vercelloni L. La tavola imbandita, storia estetica della cucina. Roma-Bari: Laterza; 2001.
Meglio L. Sociologia del cibo e dell'alimentazione. Milano: FrancoAngeli; 2012.
Moir HC. Some observations on the appreciation of flavour in foodstuffs. J Chem Technol Biotechnol. 1936;55(8):145–8.
Montanari M. Il mondo in cucina. Roma-Bari: Laterza; 2002.
Montanari M. Il cibo come cultura. Roma-Bari: Laterza; 2004.
Montanari M. Il riposo della polpetta. Roma-Bari: Laterza; 2009.
Morrot G, Brochet F, Dubourdieu D. The color of odors. Brain Lang. 2001;79:309–20.
Peters T. Quando il silenzio parla. Roma: Edizioni Paoline; 2011.
Peynaud E. Le goit du vin. Paris: Dunod; 1980.
Rebora G. La civiltà della forchetta. Roma-Bari: Laterza; 1998.
Sercambi G. Il novelliere. Roma: Salerno Editrice; 1974.
Standage T. Una storia del mondo in sei bicchieri. Torino: Codice Edizioni; 2005.

Dysphagia in Adulthood and the Geriatric Age

2

"Dysphagia" is a term derived from Greek and is composed of *fàghein*, "to eat," and the prefix *dis-*, which indicates a disorder. In short, the word "dysphagia" means "eating disorder." In clinical practice, disorders in this area have certain characteristics and consequently more complex definitions. The medical dictionary (Thomas 1993) identifies five forms of dysphagia:

1. *Constricta*: narrowing at the level of the pharynx or esophagus
2. *Lusoria*: compression of the esophagus by the right subclavian artery
3. *Oropharyngeal*: difficulty in propelling the bolus from the mouth to the esophagus
4. *Paralytic*: paralysis of the muscles of the mouth, pharynx or esophagus
5. *Spastic*: spasm of the pharynx or esophagus

In the *International Classification of Diseases* (ICD), developed by the World Health Organization (WHO), swallowing disorders are grouped under codes 787.2 (ICD-9) and R13.1 (ICD-10). In this latest version (ICD-10), they are further classified as follows:

- R13.11: dysphagia of the oral phase
- R13.12: dysphagia of the oropharyngeal phase
- R13.13: dysphagia of the pharyngeal phase
- R13.14: dysphagia of the pharyngoesophageal phase
- R13.19: other dysphagias

The most common form is oropharyngeal dysphagia, which is a disorder in one of the phases of swallowing. This process is divided by most authors into three phases: oral, pharyngeal, and esophageal. Other authors also include the preoral and gastric phases of swallowing.

A. Amitrano, *Dysphagia and Nutrition*,
https://doi.org/10.1007/978-3-031-77449-2_2

Dysphagia is not a disease but rather a symptom (Schindler 1990). This means that dysphagia is not a nosographic entity in itself but rather a manifestation of diseases that can affect systems even anatomically distant from each other (Table 2.1). Dysphagia can therefore be a symptom or a sign: it is a symptom when reported by

Table 2.1 Causes of dysphagia

Etiology	Pathological pictures
Iatrogenic	Effects of pharmacological therapies (chemotherapy, neuroleptics, etc.), head/neck surgical interventions, neurosurgical interventions Corrosive radiotherapy
Infectious	Diphtheria Botulism Lyme disease Syphilis Mucositis
Metabolic	Amyloidosis Cushing's syndrome Thyrotoxicosis Wilson's disease
Myopathic	Connective tissue diseases Dermatomyositis Myasthenia gravis Myotonic dystrophy Oculopharyngeal dystrophy Polymyositis Sarcoidosis Paraneoplastic syndromes
Neurological	Brainstem tumors Head trauma Stroke Cerebral palsy Guillain-Barré syndrome Huntington's disease Multiple sclerosis Poliomyelitis Post-polio syndrome Tardive dyskinesia Metabolic encephalopathies Amyotrophic lateral sclerosis Parkinson's disease Dementia
Structural	Cricopharyngeal bar Zenker's diverticulum Cervical scars Oropharyngeal tumors Osteophytes and skeletal anomalies Congenital malformations

the patient himself, a sign when detected by the clinician who performs the analysis (Box 2.1).

Box 2.1 Clinical Semiotics

Semiotics (from the Greek *seméion*, meaning "sign," and the suffix *-iké*, "related to") is the study of the signs of various diseases aimed at diagnosis. In medicine:

- Symptoms are subjective sensations (dyspnea, pain, nausea, etc.) reported by the patient and are to be considered true, even if they cannot be demonstrated.
- Signs are objective findings detectable by the clinician or, sometimes, by the patient himself (fever, skin lesions, hyperemia, etc.).

The two definitions—symptoms and signs—intersect with each other in a very significant way, and the division between the two types of elements is of little relevance for practical purposes. In any case, from a practical point of view, the symptom is the pure detection of the presence of an alteration that must be interpreted as a sign by the action of the clinician.

There are numerous ways in which dysphagia can manifest itself. The most common and explanatory sign is coughing, which indicates the accidental passage of food substances or internal fluids (secretions or regurgitations) into the respiratory tract. Coughing is not the only sign that can reveal a swallowing disorder but also choking, changes in voice quality after eating, the feeling of persistence of the bolus in the throat, drooling, odynophagia, weight loss, and dehydration. Dysphagia can be a sign of different pathologies:

- Neurological diseases
- Progressive disease
- Rheumatic diseases
- Connective tissue diseases
- Tumors of the organs of the alimentary tract
- Iatrogenic causes
- Respiratory disorders
- Psychiatric and psychological disorders

Dysphagia can be roughly defined as difficulty in progressing food in the swallowing tract or the erroneous direction of the bolus that accidentally starts toward the respiratory channel instead of the swallowing channel. Clinically, the two dysfunctions can present separately or in association and can be present at various levels of severity. In the most severe cases, the two processes generate malnutrition and/or aspiration pneumonia. Swallowing is a dynamic process that unfolds over time and varies according to the type of bolus that is swallowed.

This means that people may not show signs or symptoms of dysphagia with every swallowing act and especially manifest different swallowing difficulties depending on the consistency of the food they consume. It is quite common for patients with neurogenic dysphagia to have greater difficulty consuming liquid foods rather than creamy or solid foods. Conversely, in other patients, swallowing difficulties may manifest mainly when solid foods are consumed in the presence of a good ability to swallow liquid boluses. In some cases, dysphagic subjects may not show dysfunctions at the level of the musculature that determines the swallowing act but may have an insufficient state of alertness to activate safe and efficient swallowing acts. In other cases, behavioral disorders can interfere with the implementation of efficient and safe swallowing acts. Dysphagia can therefore be the consequence of not only a deficit in the swallowing musculature but also an impairment of this musculature due to external factors. Tanner (2006) defines dysphagia as a disorder of the emotional, cognitive, sensory, and/or motor acts involved in the transfer of a substance from the mouth to the stomach, which causes dehydration and malnutrition and carries the risk of choking and aspiration. Dysphagia can be distinguished from feeding disorders, which are an impediment in the process of transferring food from the outside to the mouth. In particular, a feeding disorder can be determined by a disorder or difficulty in the movements of the hands and arms that are used to bring food to the mouth. In the English-speaking world, feeding disorders and swallowing disorders, especially in the pediatric field, often overlap. Furthermore, dysphagia must be distinguished from eating disorders, such as anorexia and bulimia, which rarely present as swallowing disorders (Barofsky and Fontaine 1998). However, swallowing disorders and psychiatric disorders often find an area of contiguity that is often difficult for clinicians to disentangle. This is also due to the persistent lack of clear terminology regarding disorders in this area (Spadola et al. 2016a, b).

2.1 Incidence and Prevalence of Dysphagia

Dysphagia is a very widespread problem, although defining an exact estimate of its prevalence is difficult because of the different definitions used in various countries, the different settings in which the problem is detected, and the non-uniform use of tools for detecting swallowing problems. Dysphagia is a problem largely related to the advancement of age; it is therefore intuitive that the dimensions of the problem are somehow linked to the demographic trends of societies or, at least, to Western societies, where there is a more marked aging of the population (United Nations 2019). From 2007 to 2019, the world population increased by 1 billion, reaching 7.7 billion people.

Compared with that in 1990, the average life expectancy in the world has reached 72.6 years, increasing by approximately 9 years. People over 65 are the fastest growing social group worldwide. In 2018, for the first time in history, people over 65 outnumbered children under 5. In 2020, there were 727 million people over 65, with a projection to double by 2050, when 1.5 billion people over 65 are expected.

The percentage of elderly people, who, in 2020, represented 9.3% of the entire global social body, will increase to 16% by 2050, when one in six inhabitants will be over 65 (United Nations 2020).

Notably this age group was most affected by COVID-19, whose mortality is also related to the level of medical care and the previous health status of individuals.

Many researchers have studied the prevalence of dysphagia in different care settings. Some of them report a prevalence of dysphagia ranging from 16% to 22% in elderly communities (Bloem et al. 1990; Lindgren and Janzon 1991). A systematic review reported a 15% prevalence of dysphagia in housing communities for the elderly (Madhavan et al. 2016). In a study conducted on 211 patients in a geriatric ward in Singapore, the authors reported a prevalence of dysphagia in 29% of the sample at admission and 28% at discharge (Lee et al. 1999). The prevalence of swallowing and feeding disorders detected in a nursing home in Maryland was 60% (Siebens et al. 1986). Substantially overlapping data are reported in studies that analyze the prevalence of dysphagia in nursing homes for the elderly in other countries, such as Spain, Portugal, and South Korea (Silveira Guijarro et al. 2011; Nogueira and Reis 2013; Park et al. 2013). There are different data on the prevalence of dysphagia during hospitalization in general acute hospitals reported in the literature. In one study, Layne et al. (1989) reported the presence of swallowing disorders in one-third of hospitalized patients. The percentage of patients with dysphagia reported by Grother and Bukatman (1986) is significantly different; similar work revealed that dysphagia was present in 13% of hospitalized patients. This discrepancy in the data is related to the different definitions of dysphagia used by the authors.

In Layne's study, all patients with dehydration were classified as dysphagic. In an acute rehabilitation setting, the prevalence of dysphagia in hospitalized patients was one-third (Cherney 1994). Among the patients with dysphagia, approximately half had stroke outcomes, 20% had cranial-encephalic trauma, 7% had spinal injuries and brain tumors, and 5% had degenerative neurological diseases (ibid). Dysphagia is a very common symptom in patients with stroke. Each year, approximately 15 million people worldwide suffer a stroke, of which approximately 6 million die and another 5 million suffer disability (WHO 2014a).

Swallowing difficulties are a common comorbidity, assessed in 37%–78% of stroke patients (Martino et al. 2005). The incidence of dysphagia is highest immediately after a stroke and tends to decrease in the first few days, with percentages ranging from 51% on day zero to 27% on day seven (Smithard et al. 1997). Dysphagia seriously jeopardizes the survival of the individual, both because of the risk of choking and the possibility of passing part of the bolus into the lower airways, with a risk of developing pneumonia and ingesting triple that of patients who do not present swallowing disorders (Martino et al. 2005).

The onset of pneumonia can lead to a tripled risk of mortality for dysphagic patients (Katzan et al. 2003). Dysphagia also causes malnutrition and dehydration (Foley et al. 2009) and makes oral therapy problematic. Notably, half of the patients with post-stroke dysphagia are unaware of their swallowing problems (Parker et al. 2004).

In 59% of patients with neoplastic diseases of the head-neck district undergoing surgery and/or radiochemotherapy, signs of dysphagia are present (Pauloski et al. 2000), which, in 33%, are also detected 2 years after such treatments (Hillman et al. 1998). Dysphagia is a common symptom in patients with head trauma. The incidence reported in different studies varies from 4.5% to 78% (Field and Weiss 1989; Yorkstone et al. 1989; Howle et al. 2014; Lee et al. 2016). The considerable variability is justifiable with the different severities of head trauma and with the different evaluation tools and definitions of dysphagia used by the authors. Lazarus and Logemann reported signs of dysphagia in approximately 50% of the subjects studied via videofluoroscopic examination (Lazarus and Logemann 1987). Winstein (1983) reported that in a sample of subjects with head trauma evaluated at a rehabilitation center, 27% experienced dysphagia at admission, and 6% experienced dysphagia after 5 months of rehabilitative intervention. Yorkstone et al. (1989) reported that 13% of patients remain dysphagic after head injury.

Dysphagia is a very common symptom of neurological progressive diseases, such as Parkinson's disease, amyotrophic lateral sclerosis (ALS), multiple sclerosis (MS), and myasthenia gravis. Under these neurological conditions, dysphagia, which has a variable onset, is not stable and generally tends to worsen as the disease progresses. This aspect should be considered as an additional difficulty in prevalence studies, in which the data can differ significantly, depending on the stages of the disease in which the symptom of dysphagia is detected. The incidence and prevalence of Parkinson's disease vary from 18% to 100% (Bird et al. 1994; Clarke et al. 1998; Miller 1999; Potulska et al. 2003; Bakke et al. 2011). Many authors agree that dysphagia is a symptom found in 50% of sick individuals (Lieberman et al. 1980; Edwards et al. 1991; Bushmann et al. 1989). Suttrup and Warnecke (2016) reported that 80% of those affected by Parkinson's disease develop dysphagia during the entire progression of the disease. Some authors report the early onset of swallowing disorders in patients with Parkinson's disease (Robbins et al. 1986; Sung et al. 2010).

Although the relationship between the severity of motor symptoms and dysphagia is not clear, it is generally accepted that the severity of dysphagia increases as other symptoms worsen (Robbins et al. 1986; Ali et al. 1996; Fuh et al. 1997; Monte et al. 2005). However, it is important to emphasize that even in the early stages of the disease, severe swallowing disorders can be detected. Moreover, the prevalence of dysphagia is greater in patients with Parkinson's disease who have a significant degree of cognitive decline (Bine et al. 1995). In amyotrophic lateral sclerosis, dysphagia can be one of the onset symptoms of the pathology itself, especially in the bulbar form. Some studies report that between 25% and 30% of patients with ALS show signs of bulbar symptomatology at the first diagnosis (Mulder 1980; Caroscio et al. 1987). This means that approximately one-third of patients have swallowing disorders from the onset of the disease. The progression of ALS inevitably leads to an increase in the severity of dysphagia (Hillel and Miller 1989; Fattori et al. 2006). Further studies have highlighted episodes of silent aspiration during swallowing in 58% of patients with ALS (Plowman et al. 2016).

In multiple sclerosis, Hartelius and Svensson (1994) reported that approximately 33% of patients have problems with chewing and swallowing. Patients with MS, followed by outpatients during *follow-up*, present with a percentage of dysphagia ranging from 30% to 40% (Restivo et al. 2006). In a study of 143 patients, Calcagno et al. (2002) reported signs of dysphagia in 34% of the sample. The severity of dysphagia increases with the progression of the disease, affecting approximately 65% of patients with MS (De Pauw et al. 2002).

Approximately one-third of patients with myasthenia gravis have swallowing disorders (Llabrés et al. 2005). The prevalence of dysphagia largely depends on the extent of muscle fatigue and the degree of impairment of the respiratory muscles (Murray 1962).

Dysphagia is a symptom of rheumatic diseases. Oh et al. (2007) reported the presence of signs of dysphagia in 62 of the 738 studied subjects with polymyositis and dermatomyositis. Cases of dysphagia are reported in patients with inclusion body myositis (Zeng and Schmidt 2020). Symptoms of dysphagia are also reported in patients with rheumatoid arthritis (Geterud et al. 1991; Ekberg et al. 1987; Erb et al. 2001). Ninety percent of patients with scleroderma have disorders, mainly in the esophageal phase of swallowing (Fulp and Castell 1990; Ntoumazios et al. 2006). Approximately 65–75% of patients with Sjögren's syndrome have dysphagia (Grande et al. 1993; Mandl et al. 2007). The prevalence of swallowing difficulties in patients with dementia varies from 13% to 57%. Dysphagia is present during the final stages of frontotemporal dementia (FTD) but has also been observed during the initial phase of Alzheimer's disease (AD) (Alagiakrishnan et al. 2013). Dysphagia is also a common symptom in individuals with developmental disabilities, despite the limited number of studies investigating the prevalence of swallowing disorders in this particular population, which Leslie et al. (2008) define as the *Cinderella population*. In fact, compared with several studies that analyze the incidence and prevalence rates in other population groups, the literature provides only a few studies with a broad view of swallowing problems in individuals with developmental disabilities. This lack of data can result in insufficient planning of services for the management of swallowing problems in this particular social group. Importantly, respiratory infections are the cause of death in 52% of adults with developmental disabilities (Hollins et al. 1998). The estimate of the spread of swallowing problems in individuals with developmental disabilities varies from 36% (Hickman 1997) to 73% (Rogers et al. 1994). Dysphagia is a symptom found in approximately 60% of individuals with cerebral palsy (Eyman et al. 1990; Chadwick et al. 2002). These studies also reported the presence of dysphagia in individuals with Down syndrome, with or without dementia, and in individuals with severe developmental disabilities. Jackson et al. (2016) studied a cohort of 138 individuals with Down syndrome and reported swallowing disorders in the oral phase in 65% of the sample and in the pharyngeal phase with aspiration in 56%.

2.2 The Consequences of Dysphagia

Dysphagia limits a patient's health consequences for a patient's health, and in the most severe cases, it can endanger survival, influence nutritional status, and create risk situations, such as choking and aspiration pneumonia (*ab ingestis*), due to the passage of a bolus into the airways (Mandell and Niederman 2019). Dysphagia limits a patient's health ability to carry out normal daily activities and significantly impacts quality of life, which negatively affects the entire family group; one of the aspects of food is caregiving, which is inevitably lacking in severely dysphagic individuals, for whom any form of oral feeding is impossible. Dysphagia is considered a real mourning, both for the individual who suffers from it and for the family group to which they belong (Amitrano 2019), and has a significant effect on rehabilitation times, on the need for care and assistance, and, therefore, ultimately, on the costs for health services. Therefore, the consequences of dysphagia include increases in morbidity, mortality, and health costs (WHO 2014b; Maeshima et al. 2011; Guyomard et al. 2009; Altman et al. 2010).

2.2.1 Malnutrition

The term "malnutrition" refers to a "state of functional, structural, and developmental alteration of the organism, resulting from a discrepancy between specific nutritional needs and intake or utilization of essential nutrients" (*Council on Food and Nutrition of the American Medical Association*). Malnutrition can occur at various levels in relation to body mass index (BMI) (Table 2.2).

The assessment of nutritional status is a complex procedure that must be carried out by specialized professionals. The diagnosis of malnutrition is based on the data from the patient's history, physical examination, and laboratory test results. One of the most important indicators of malnutrition or risk of malnutrition is the assessment of changes in body weight in the months prior to observation. An unintended body weight loss of 5% in the last month or 10% in the last 3 months is strongly indicative of malnutrition. Protein-calorie malnutrition has a significant effect on patient prognosis. Malnourished subjects have a higher mortality, a higher incidence of complications, and prolonged hospital stays, as well as a noticeable worsening of quality of life (Riso et al. 2001). Patients with swallowing disorders often experience changes in nutritional status caused by a decrease in intake. There is a close correlation between the severity of dysphagia and the incidence of malnutrition (Clavé et al. 2006). However, several factors, such as the prevalence of malnutrition among patients with dysphagia and the pathophysiology of associated malnutrition, are not yet well understood. Notably malnutrition is a predictor of the onset of sarcopenia (Beaudart et al. 2019), that is, the progressive decline in muscle mass and strength, which is mainly due to the aging of the human body. Recently,

Table 2.2 Levels of malnutrition

Severe malnutrition	BMI <16
Moderate malnutrition	BMI 16–16.9
Mild malnutrition	BMI 17–18.4
Normal weight	BMI 18.5–24.9
Overweight	BMI 25–29.9
Obesity	BMI ≥30

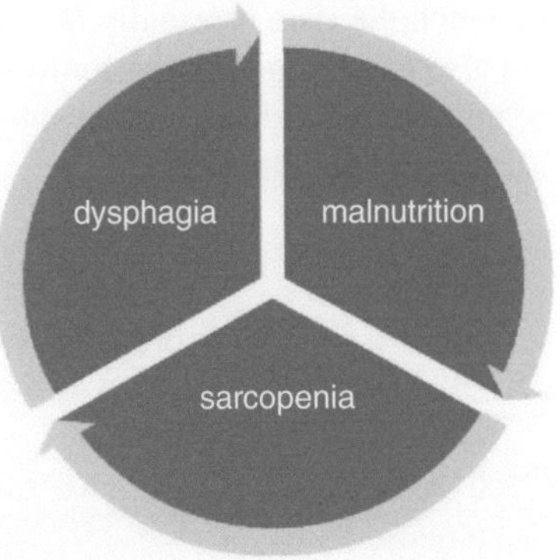

Fig. 2.1 Circulatory process: dysphagia-malnutrition-sarcopenia

the concept of "sarcopenic dysphagia," that is, difficulty swallowing due to sarcopenia of the swallowing muscles, was introduced (Wakabayashi 2014). In such cases, a circular process is established that sees dysphagia as the cause of malnutrition, which, in turn, determines that sarcopenia is capable of contributing to further worsening of the initial dysphagia (Fig. 2.1): a circular dysfunctional process to be interrupted with appropriate rehabilitative procedures.

2.2.2 The Passage of a Food Bolus into the Airways

Among the main consequences of dysphagia, we must consider the accidental passage of a food bolus into the airways. Indeed, the normal physiology of swallowing is based on the delicate balance of respiratory and feeding functions, which, at least in the first part of their journey within the human body, share the same anatomical structures. When we breathe, we do not eat, and when we eat, we do not breathe; this is the phrase by Jeri Logemann (Lazarus and Logemann 1987), which effectively summarizes how the coordination between breathing and swallowing is at the basis of the safety of the swallowing act. Some anatomical sphincters, which act as a real system of valves, alternately open the swallowing and feeding channels to prevent air from going into the swallowing channel and, vice versa, food into the respiratory channel, thus avoiding the overlap of the two functions. In some conditions related to pathology or inattention, such as sudden laughter while one is eating, dangerous situations can occur, sometimes even fatal. The entry of a food bolus into the airways can cause choking and the introduction of food into the lower airways. Choking or asphyxiation is a condition in which normal breathing is hindered owing to direct or indirect factors that prevent the correct exchange of gases with the environment. The presence of food or foreign bodies in the larynx or trachea and the aspiration of vomiting are among the direct causes of choking. Such factors, as the popular Italian saying reminds us, "When you eat you fight with death," pose a risk to everyone who eats, but it is reasonable to believe that the risk is greater in situations of swallowing dysfunction. There are no data on the risk of choking in dysphagic individuals, but epidemiological data are available for the general population, in which the risk, especially in children, is linked not only to the ingestion of food but also to the ingestion of nonfood substances. Choking is among the major causes of unintentional death among subjects under 14 years of age (Paulozzi et al. 2006; Ministry of Health 2017).

Box 2.2 Mochi

Mochi is a typical preparation of traditional Japanese cuisine. It is a food made from glutinous rice that is chopped and pounded until a soft and sticky white paste is obtained. The paste is then molded into spherical or rectangular shapes that contain a sweet or savory filling. *Mochi* is preferably consumed warm.

Some studies report that 60%–80% of food choking episodes affect the total number of choking incidents (Foltran et al. 2012). In Japan, in 2018, 4600 people died as a result of food choking (Ministry of Health, Labour and Welfare 2018). On average, in Japan from 2006 to 2016, approximately 4000 people per year died from food choking (Taniguchi et al. 2021). In this study, the most significant number of deceased people was those over 75 years old. Notably the highest number of deaths occurs in the first days of the year, which coincides with the consumption of *mochi*, the typical food of Japanese tradition, which is eaten mainly during New Year (Box 2.2).

In Europe, according to the latest available statistical surveys, on average, 500 children per year die from choking. The situation in Italy is not better. In fact, every year, at least 1000 children are hospitalized for serious cases of choking. In 2012, there were more than 718 healthy people in Italy admitted to intensive care for "bolus food" or "airway obstruction," with a tragic toll of victims: 280 deaths, of which approximately 50 were children. In 2013, in the United States, there were 5595 deaths from suffocation, which were distributed differently across various age groups (*Center for Disease Control and Prevention*) (Table 2.3).

Notably, the number of deaths from suffocation (the data also refer to the ingestion of nonfood substances) is greater in the extreme age groups, i.e., children and elderly individuals. This is also a common trend in statistics recorded in other countries. In a chart related to Italy from 1999 to 2003, it is evident that the highest number of victims is located in the extreme population groups (Fig. 2.2).

Table 2.3 Deaths from suffocation in the United States in 2013

Age	Number of deaths from suffocation
0–1	905
1–4	134
5–9	31
10–14	48
45–54	464
55–64	613
65 and over	3400

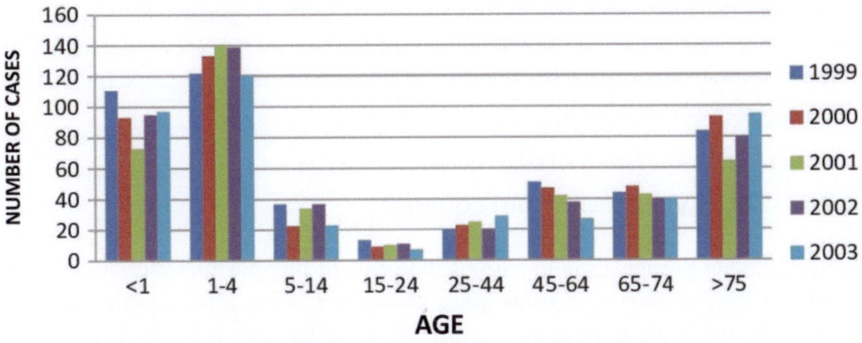

Fig. 2.2 Deaths by choking in Italy from 1999 to 2003

In not all cases does the passage of a bolus or even nonfood substances into the airways cause suffocation. Depending on the dimensions and characteristics of the bolus, slippage of the food substance into the lower airways can occur. In these cases, in the field of deglutology, the two terms "aspiration" and "penetration" are used. In fact, we speak of penetration when the bolus enters the larynx but does not pass the glottic plane and of aspiration when the bolus passes the glottic plane. Normally, the passage of a bolus into the airways triggers the cough reflex or *raclage*; when this does not happen, it is referred to as *silent aspiration*. The passage of a bolus into the airways can occur at different times during the swallowing process. Specifically, pre-*swallowing aspiratory penetration* occurs when passage in the airways occurs during the oral preparation phase, that is, before triggering the swallowing act. We discuss intra-swallowing *aspiratory penetration* when the passage occurs during the swallowing act and, finally, post-swallowing *aspiratory penetration* when it occurs at the end of the swallowing act.

The passage of a contaminated bolus into the lung cavity causes the onset of pneumonia, a potentially severe lung inflammatory condition (Marik 2001). It is important to distinguish between *aspiration pneumonia* and *aspiration pneumonitis*, both of which are consequences of the passage of substances into the lower airways. In the case of *aspiration pneumonia*, it refers to the passage of potentially contaminated oral content into the lung cavities; in the case of *aspiration pneumonitis*, the passage into the lower airways is of gastric reflux, which initially becomes sterile, although subsequent bacterial superinfection is possible. The incidence of aspiration pneumonia is not well defined due to the discrepancy, in different studies, in the definition of aspiration pneumonia used and the quality of dysphagia assessment. In different studies, the estimated percentage of aspiration pneumonia out of total pneumonia varies from 5% to 60%. The incidence of aspiration pneumonia out of total pneumonia ranges from 5% to 16.5% in Spain, France, and North America; a multicenter Japanese study reported a percentage of 60% (Mitsuhata and Teramoto 2020). The highest risk of aspiration pneumonia is found in elderly individuals with concomitant diseases and in adult individuals undergoing head-neck surgery (Manabe et al. 2015; Teramoto et al. 2009, 2015). Pneumonia is the leading cause of death in those over 65 years of age (Teramoto and Komiya 2020).

Notably the onset of aspiration pneumonia (*aspiration pneumonia*) is significantly influenced by bacterial contamination of the boluses that are aspirated; in this context, several authors have highlighted the importance of oral hygiene for prevention (Nakagawa et al. 2020).

2.2.3 The Psychosocial Consequences

Eating involves participation in various moments of life that contribute to the creation and maintenance of various kinds of social relationships. Dysphagia often leads to the isolation of the subject, who eats alone the special foods that he must consume, preferring not to disturb the diners with frequent coughing and/or for the discomfort caused by the possible poor continence of food from the lips or the presence of sialorrhea (Ekberg et al. 2002; Farri et al. 2007). Social occasions related to food, such as going to a restaurant or bar, are also avoided, as are, in some cases, taking communion at mass (Ekberg et al. 2002). In dysphagic patients, emotional reactions can also develop, such as the fear of eating. Verdonschot et al. (2016) reported signs of anxiety and depression in dysphagic patients. Specific tools, such as the SWAL-QOL and the MDADI, have been constructed to assess the impact of dysphagia on patients' quality of life. The SWAL-QOL, whose name derives from the combination of the abbreviated term *swallowing* with the acronym for *quality of life*, is designed to understand how swallowing problems affect patients' daily life (McHorney et al. 2002) through a test that contains 43 items divided into 11 sections. A group of researchers—from the Department of Head and Neck Surgery at the MD Anderson Cancer Center in Texas and the Department of Biometry at the School of Public Health at the University of Texas—developed a standardized self-assessment questionnaire called the *MD Anderson Dysphagia Inventory* (MDADI), which is specifically designed to assess the impact of dysphagia on the quality of life of patients undergoing head and neck surgery (Chen et al. 2001) and consists of 20 questions grouped into 3 domains (emotional, functional, and physical).

2.3 Clinical Management of Dysphagic Patients

The clinical management of dysphagic patients is multiprofessional and multidisciplinary. The complexity of the problem indeed requires the involvement of multiple professionals in various care settings in which the clinical management of dysphagia is articulated: acute, subacute, rehabilitation, and home care. In each of these settings, management assumes unique characteristics that involve different operators. The link between the effectiveness of the management of dysphagic patients and the efficiency of the entire care network is highly realistic. The management network must be equipped with the necessary professionals specifically trained to meet the patient's needs and to work as a team. Cooperation and coordination must be among the various professionals involved are essential to achieve the goal of feeding the patient while respecting safety and nutritional adequacy criteria. In some centers, mainly overseas, a *swallowing team* coordinated by the *swallowing team leader* (Groher and Crary 2021) is present and active within the institutions that care for patients with dysphagia.

The management of patients with dysphagia can be divided into three major areas: evaluation, re-education, and routine management. The evaluation is the first essential moment of taking charge of the case and serves *primarily* to detect the presence of the problem and then to identify the pathophysiological mechanisms that determine it, thus allowing the establishment of the methods and objectives of rehabilitative treatment. The re-educational phase is the one in which remedial or compensatory procedures are implemented, which is useful for allowing the patient to achieve functional swallowing. Routine management occurs both during the rehabilitative process and at the end of it and concerns patients who can eat orally, even with special precautions. In this phase, caregivers and those who take care of food preparation and the management of *mealtime* play a fundamental role.

2.3.1 Professionals Involved in the Management of Patients with Dysphagia

Depending on the severity and needs of the patient, various professionals are involved in the clinical management of dysphagic patients, each with their own specificity (Fig. 2.3). The key role in our country is played by the phoniatrician and the speech therapist, both of which are involved in all care settings. However, many of the professionals involved differ in their involvement, depending on the phase of the clinical path in which the patient is taken care of, the specific professional, and the organization of health services in various realities. In the medical field, phoniatricians, otolaryngologists, neurologists, pneumologists, nutritionists, radiologists, physiatrists, gastroenterologists, thoracic surgeons, child neuropsychiatrists, and

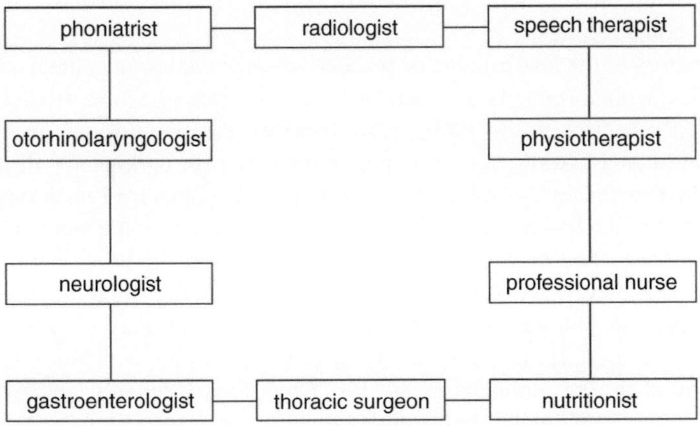

Fig. 2.3 Professionals involved in the management of dysphagia. (Source: courtesy of Professor Giovanni Ruoppolo)

Fig. 2.4 Roles in the management of dysphagia. (Source: courtesy of Professor Giovanni Ruoppolo)

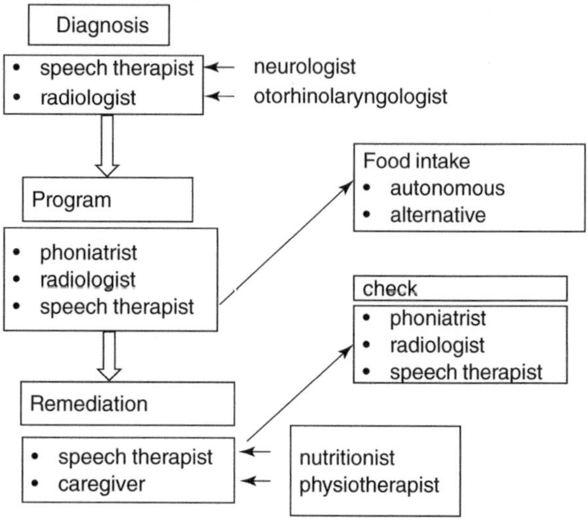

dentists are involved. Among the nonmedical health personnel, speech therapists, nurses, physiotherapists, respiratory physiotherapists, occupational therapists, dietitians, nurses, dental hygienists, and psychologists are involved. The role of health assistants, caregivers in general, and kitchen staff, who are engaged in food preparation and assistance daily during meals, is also significant. Not all the professionals mentioned here, whose rich list is probably incomplete compared with specific local organizations and the specific needs of some patients, are necessarily engaged simultaneously, but their involvement varies depending on the patient's age group and the swallowing problems presented (Fig. 2.4).

In all phases of the clinical path of dysphagic patients, the speech-language therapist plays a central role. In many American hospitals, the speech-language therapist is the *swallowing team leader* (Groher and Crary 2021). The speech therapist is present in the management of patients in acute, subacute, rehabilitative, and home settings.

The history of the involvement of speech-language therapists in the management of patients with dysphagia is relatively long. In fact, the first studies by Jeri Logemann date back to the 1960s, who identified videofluoroscopy as a suitable technique to study swallowing function in subjects with Parkinson's disease. Her studies then moved on to swallowing in patients undergoing head-neck surgery, and in 1976, one of the first papers on the subject was presented at the national congress of the American Speech-Language-Hearing Association. In 1974, George Larsen published the first work written by a speech-language therapist on the management of dysphagia in patients with neurological diseases. In Italy, Oskar Schindler (Ruoppolo et al. 2021) introduced the scientific discipline of deglutology, which was born with the publication of his *Operational Manual of Swallowing Pathophysiology* (Schindler 1990). Rehabilitation for dysphagia is an activity that involves an increasing number of speech therapists. The speech-language therapist involved in the evaluation and rehabilitation of dysphagic patients must have both adequate specific training and extensive experience in the evaluation and treatment of patients with swallowing disorders (ASHA 2002b). It is therefore necessary for deglutologist speech therapists to have proper clinical, technical, communicative, interprofessional, and transcultural skills. In fact, the need to relate to more different professional figures than those with whom he usually collaborates requires knowledge of new areas for mutual respect of professional skills. Moreover, the increasing presence of citizens belonging to different religions and cultures requires deglutologist speech therapists to understand traditions, especially food taboos, in other cultures. This is due to the strong influence that culture has on food and consequently on swallowing.

2.3.2 Different Care Settings for Dysphagic Patients

In the acute phase, speech therapy intervention aims to assess swallowing difficulties and to determine whether the patient should be fed *orally*, taking into account safety and nutritional adequacy. It is essential, especially in patients with risk factors, to evaluate their swallowing ability before resuming feeding. In patients where it is possible to maintain oral *mouth*-feeding, the most suitable method is identified. Whenever possible, mouth-feeding is identified as the most suitable method, where it is necessary to modify the food textures and pay particular attention to the posture to be maintained during the meal. In this phase, which is still highly unstable, starting real rehabilitation treatment is difficult, even when necessary. Thus, most of the time, rehabilitation care inevitably focuses on identifying the most suitable compensatory interventions. Additionally, in this phase of great instability, it is necessary to monitor the patient and modify the decisions made on the basis of the results of the most recent assessment. In the subacute phase, when the patient is more stable, it is necessary to continue monitoring swallowing function, and often, at this stage, starting a real rehabilitation program may be possible. Attention to the kind of foods and the postures adopted by the patient during mealtime continues to be of greatest importance at this stage. Notably, in the first two phases, the acute and subacute phases, of the clinical path, the patient generally consumes his meals while staying in bed. The intake of food while in bed requires particular care to avoid possible risk situations. The patient must eat with the back of the bed raised to 90°, and as a precautionary measure, support should be placed behind the neck to prevent the head from being extended. It is also useful to slightly raise the lower part of the bed to slightly flex the knees. In this way, for the patient, it is easier to maintain the sitting position during the entire meal, preventing him from slowly sliding down. Importantly, the patient, especially if spoon-fed, must keep his gaze fixed in front of him without rotating his head to meet the spoon. In fact, head movements modify the progression of the bolus in the swallowing channel, which is why the posture of the head held during a meal may not guarantee safety. Finally, if the patient is unable to feed himself, the caregiver should be educated on the correct methods to perform this operation. In fact, when a patient who is in bed is fed, his head is likely to slide into an extended position, thus increasing the risk of aspiration. In the rehabilitation phase, in those patients in which symptoms of dysphagia are still present, actual rehabilitation treatment begins on the basis of the results of the evaluation and with tools and methods that rehabilitative practice has particularly enriched in recent years. In home settings, the speech-language therapist is faced with clinical problems that are not different from those of the hospitalized patient. In this case, both the evaluative and rehabilitative works differ because the environmental patient context itself is different. In fact, if the institution guarantees, at least theoretically, a uniform environment, the home environment is extremely variable. This increases in a varying and not predetermined way the complexity of patient care. Greater caution is needed, both in the execution of feeding tests and in the execution of functional stimulation with boluses that can cause choking, owing to the immediate unavailability of support offered by the hospital network.

The intervention, especially the rehabilitative intervention, must be adapted to the context in which the patient is hospitalized. The adaptation of the characteristics of the home environment to the needs of dysphagic patients is essential. Particular care must be given to the meal setting, where, if necessary, adapted dishes will be adopted, a suitable seat provided, and possibly all distraction factors eliminated. It is also important to train nonprofessional caregivers about the management and assistance of the meals of patients with dysphagia. Finally, regarding the management of such a patient, it is useful to remember that national and international guidelines are now available to clinicians, which drive clinical practice according to the principles of *evidence-based medicine* (EBM). Many health facilities have also equipped themselves with diagnostic therapeutic care pathways (PDTAs) for dysphagia. In Italy, it is worth remembering the PDTA of dysphagia in the Piedmont Region, published in 2013 (Regional Agency for Health Services—Piedmont Region 2013).

2.4 Speech Therapy Management of Patients with Dysphagia

Speech therapy for patients with dysphagia consists of two main phases: evaluation and treatment. The evaluation (ref. CAP. 3) is the first and essential moment of care. In fact, in this phase, the presence of the swallowing problem is identified, and its dysfunctional mechanisms are outlined. In our country, unlike other realities, speech-language therapists perform only clinical evaluation. This, in some contexts, can provide exhaustive answers to a certain extent, whereas in other cases, an instrumental evaluation may be needed. If the clinical assessment fails to provide an adequate explanation of the patient's symptoms, if silent aspiration is suspected, or if a more in-depth visualization of the various phases of swallowing is needed, instrumental evaluation is used (Groher and Crary 2021). The American Speech-Language-Hearing Association (ASHA) has published clinical indicators for instrumental evaluation (ASHA 2002a). The evaluation also serves to monitor the evolution of the swallowing disorder and to document progress and the results of rehabilitation. The ability to evaluate the swallowing behavior of the patient is an essential skill for the speech therapist, who finds himself daily in the condition of monitoring the patient's performance both to establish the progression of the rehabilitation program and to graduate the level of individual exercise (ASHA 2002b). Importantly, caregivers can also monitor patient's swallowing behaviour to avoid being fed per os patients in conditions not suitable for the safety of the meal. The evaluation of swallowing functionality remains a delicate activity and is exclusive to the health professionals in charge, who have a high level of preparation and specific experience. However, other operators involved in meal assistance need to be able to grasp the signs that can manifest in situations where it is risky to feed patients per os, even those for whom previously a positive indication was given in this sense. Situations of low vigilance and cooperation on the part of the patient must lead to the discontinuation of feeding per os and the request of a specific evaluative intervention.

The rehabilitative phase follows the evaluation. The general purpose of treatment is to enable patients to feed themselves sufficiently, avoiding dehydration or malnutrition, without running the risk of choking or aspiration pneumonia. The options that can be adopted to achieve this purpose are as follows:

- Behavioral treatment
- Dietary adaptations
- Medical treatment
- Surgical treatment

Behavioral treatment includes compensation strategies that may include head postures, feeding rhythms, and rehabilitation treatments for learning new swallowing modalities or for muscle strengthening. Dietary adaptations refer to the modification of the characteristics of food on the basis of the patient's swallowing difficulties. In this sense, it may be necessary to modify the texture and taste of foods or the volume of individual boluses. Medical treatment may involve substituting, when possible, drugs that have a negative impact on the patient's mental and swallowing state. In some cases, it may be necessary to place a nasogastric tube (NGT) to provide nutrition to the patient if the data from the evaluation advise against feeding per os. Surgical treatment may be necessary in some clinical situations or for the placement of percutaneous gastrostomy (PEG). The treatment options mentioned should not be considered alternatives, but resorting to multiple modes of intervention at the same time is very common.

References

Alagiakrishnan K, Bhanji RA, Kurian M. Evaluation and management of oropharyngeal dysphagia in different types of dementia: a systematic review. Arch Gerontol Geriatr. 2013;56(1):1–9. https://doi.org/10.1016/j.archger.2012.04.011.

Ali GN, Wallace KL, Schwartz R, DeCarle DJ, Zagami AS, Cook IJ. Mechanisms of oral-pharyngeal dysphagia in patients with Parkinson's disease. Gastroenterology. 1996;110(2):383–92. https://doi.org/10.1053/gast.1996.v110.pm8566584.

Altman KW, Yu GP, Schaefer SD. Consequence of dysphagia in the hospitalized patient: impact on prognosis and hospital resources. Arch Otolaryngol Head Neck Surg. 2010;136(8):784–9.

Amitrano A. Dysphagia as mourning. Italian J Palliative Care. 2019;21(1):46–50.

ASHA (American Speech-Language-Hearing Association). Clinical indicators for instrumental assessment of dysphagia: guidelines, desk reference. Rockville Pike: ASHA; 2002a.

ASHA (American Speech-Language-Hearing Association). Knowledge and skills for speech-language pathologist providing service to individuals with swallowing and/or feeding disorders. Rockville Pike: ASHA Suppl; 2002b. p. 22–81.

Bakke M, Larsen SL, Lautrup C, Karlsborg M. Orofacial function and oral health in patients with Parkinson's disease. Eur J Oral Sci. 2011;119(1):27–32. https://doi.org/10.1111/j.1600-0722.2010.00802.x.

Barofsky I, Fontaine KR. Do psychogenic dysphagia patients have an eating disorder? Dysphagia. 1998;13:24.

Beaudart C, Sanchez-Rodriguez D, Locquet M, Reginster JY, Lengelé L, Bruyère O. Malnutrition as a strong predictor of the onset of sarcopenia. Nutrients. 2019;11(12):2883. https://doi.org/10.3390/nu11122883.

Bine JE, Frank EM, Mc DH, L. Dysphagia and dementia in subjects with Parkinson's disease. Dysphagia. 1995;10:160.

Bird MR, Woodward MC, Gibson EM, Phyland DJ, Fonda D. Asymptomatic swallowing disorders in elderly patients with Parkinson's disease: a description of findings on clinical examination and videofluoroscopy in sixteen patients. Age Ageing. 1994;23(3):251–4. https://doi.org/10.1093/ageing/23.3.251.

Bloem BR, Lagaay AM, van Beek W, Haan J, Roos RA, Wintzen AR. Prevalence of subjective dysphagia in community residents aged over 87. BMJ. 1990;300(6726):721–2. https://doi.org/10.1136/bmj.300.6726.

Bushmann M, Dobmeyer SM, Leeker L, Perlmutter JS. Swallowing abnormalities and their response to treatment in Parkinson's disease. Neurology. 1989;39(10):1309–14. https://doi.org/10.1212/wnl.39.10.1309.

Calcagno P, Ruoppolo G, Grasso MG, De Vincentiis M, Paolucci S. Dysphagia in multiple sclerosis—prevalence and prognostic factors. Acta Neurol Scand. 2002;105(1):40–3. https://doi.org/10.1034/j.1600-0404.2002.10062.x.

Caroscio JT, Mulvihill MN, Sterling R, Abrams B. Amyotrophic lateral sclerosis. Its natural history. Neurol Clin. 1987;5(1):1–8.

Chadwick D, Jolliffe J, Golbart J. Carer knowledge of dysphagia management strategies. Int J Lang Commun Disord. 2002;72:345–57.

Chen AY, Frankowshi R, Bishop-Leone J, Hebert T, Leyk S, Lewin J, Goepfert H. The development and validation of a dysphagia-specific quality-of-life questionnaire for patients with head and neck cancer: the M. D. Anderson Dysphagia Inventory. Arch Otolaryngol Head Neck Surg. 2001;127(7):870–6.

Cherney LR. Dysphagia in adults with neurologic disorders: an overview. In: Cherney LR, editor. Clinical management of dysphagia in adults and children. Gaithersburg: Aspen; 1994.

Clarke CE, Gullaksen E, Macdonald S, Lowe F. Referral criteria for speech and language therapy assessment of dysphagia caused by idiopathic Parkinson's disease. Acta Neurol Scand. 1998;97(1):27–35. https://doi.org/10.1111/j.1600-0404.1998.tb00605.x.

Clavé P, de Kraa M, Arreola V, Girvent M, Farré R, Palomera E, Serra-Prat M. The effect of bolus viscosity on swallowing function in neurogenic dysphagia. Aliment Pharmacol Ther. 2006;24(9):1385–94. https://doi.org/10.1111/j.1365-2036.2006.03118.x.

Edwards LL, Pfeiffer RF, Quigley EMM, Hofman R, Balluff M. Gastrointestinal symptoms in Parkinson's disease. Mov Disord. 1991;6(2):151–6.

Ekberg O, Redlund-Johnell I, Sjöblom KG. Pharyngeal function in patients with rheumatoid arthritis of the cervical spine and temporomandibular joint. Acta Radiol. 1987;28(1):35–9.

Ekberg O, Hamdy S, Woisard V, Wuttge-Hannig A, Ortega P. Social and psychological burden of dysphagia: its impact on diagnosis and treatment. Dysphagia. 2002;17(2):139–46. https://doi.org/10.1007/s00455-001-0113-5.

Erb N, Pace AV, Delamere JP, Kitas GD. Dysphagia and stridor caused by laryngeal rheumatoid arthritis. Rheumatology (Oxford). 2001;40(8):952–3. https://doi.org/10.1093/rheumatology/40.8.952.

Eyman RK, Grossman HJ, Chaney RH, Call TL. The life expectancy of profoundly handicapped people with mental retardation. N Engl J Med. 1990;323(9):584–9. https://doi.org/10.1056/NEJM199008303230906.

Farri A, Accornero A, Burdese C. Social importance of dysphagia: its impact on diagnosis and therapy. Acta Otorhinolaryngol Ital. 2007;27(2):83–6.

Fattori B, Grosso M, Bongioanni P, Nacci A, Cristofani R, AlSharif A, Licitra R, Matteucci F, Rossi B, Rubello D, Ursino F, Mariani G. Assessment of swallowing by oropharyngoesophageal scintigraphy in patients with amyotrophic lateral sclerosis. Dysphagia. 2006;21(4):280–6. https://doi.org/10.1007/s00455-006-9052-5.

Field LH, Weiss CJ. Dysphagia with head injury. Brain Inj. 1989;3(1):19–26.

Foley NC, Martin RE, Salter KL, Teasell RW. A review of the relationship between dysphagia and malnutrition following stroke. J Rehabil Med. 2009;41(9):707–13. https://doi.org/10.2340/16501977-0415.

Foltran F, Ballali S, Passali FM, Kern E, Morra B, Passali GC, Berchialla P, Lauriello M, Gregori D. Foreign bodies in the airways: a meta-analysis of published papers. Int J Pediatr Otorhinolaryngol. 2012 May;14(76 Suppl 1):S12–9. https://doi.org/10.1016/j.ijporl.2012.02.004.

Fuh JL, Lee RC, Wang SJ, Lin CH, Wang PN, Chiang JH, Liu HC. Swallowing difficulty in Parkinson's disease. Clin Neurol Neurosurg. 1997;99(2):106–12. https://doi.org/10.1016/s0303-8467(97)00606-9.

Fulp SR, Castell DO. Scleroderma esophagus. Dysphagia. 1990;5(4):204–10.

Geterud A, Bake B, Bjelle A, Jonsson R, Sandberg N, Ejnell H. Swallowing problems in rheumatoid arthritis. Acta Otolaryngol. 1991;111(6):1153–61. https://doi.org/10.3109/00016489109100771.

Grande L, Lacima G, Ros E, Font J, Pera C. Esophageal motor function in primary Sjögren's syndrome. Am J Gastroenterol. 1993;88(3):378–81.

Groher ME, Crary MA. Dysphagia clinical management in adults and children. St. Louis: Elsevier; 2021.

Grother ME, Bukatman R. The prevalence of swallowing disorders in two teaching hospitals. Dysphagia. 1986;1:3–6.

Guyomard V, Fulcher RA, Redmayne O, Metcalf AK, Potter JF, Myint PK. Effect of dysphasia and dysphagia on inpatient mortality and hospital length of stay: a database study. J Am Geriatr Soc. 2009;57(11):2101–6. https://doi.org/10.1111/j.1532-5415.2009.02526.x.

Hartelius L, Svensson P. Speech and swallowing symptoms associated with Parkinson's disease and multiple sclerosis: a survey. Folia Phoniatr Logop. 1994;46(1):9–17.

Hickman J. ALD and dysphagia: issue and practice. Speech Lang Ther Pract. 1997;1997:8–11.

Hillel AD, Miller R. Bulbar amyotrophic lateral sclerosis: patterns of progression and clinical management. Head Neck. 1989;11(1):51–9.

Hillman RE, Walsh MJ, Wolf GT, Fisher SG, Hong WK. Functional outcomes following treatment for advanced laryngeal cancer. Part I—voice preservation in advanced laryngeal cancer. Part II—laryngectomy rehabilitation: the state of the art in the VA system. Research speech-language pathologists. Department of Veterans Affairs Laryngeal Cancer Study Group. Ann Otol Rhinol Laryngol Suppl. 1998;172:1–27.

Hollins S, Attard MT, von Fraunhofer N, McGuigan S, Sedgwick P. Mortality in people with learning disability: risks, causes, and death certification findings in London. Dev Med Child Neurol. 1998;40(1):50–6.

Howle AA, Baguley IJ, Brown L. Management of dysphagia following traumatic brain injury. Curr Phys Med Rehabil Rep. 2014;2:219–30.

Jackson A, Maybee J, Moran MK, Wolter-Warmerdam K, Hickey F. Clinical characteristics of dysphagia in children with Down syndrome. Dysphagia. 2016;31(5):663–71. https://doi.org/10.1007/s00455-016-9725-7.

Katzan IL, Cebul RD, Husak SH, Dawson NV, Baker DW. The effect of pneumonia on mortality among patients hospitalized for acute stroke. Neurology. 2003;60(4):620–5. https://doi.org/10.1212/01.wnl.0000046586.38284.60.

Layne KA, Losinski DS, Zenner PM, Ament JA. Using the Fleming index of dysphagia to establish prevalence. Dysphagia. 1989;4(1):39–42. https://doi.org/10.1007/BF02407401.

Lazarus C, Logemann JA. Swallowing disorders in close head trauma patients. Arch Phys Med Rehabil. 1987;68(2):79–84.

Lee A, Sitoh YY, Lieu PK, Phua SY, Chin JJ. Swallowing impairment and feeding dependency in the hospitalised elderly. Ann Acad Med Singap. 1999;28(3):371–6.

Lee WK, Yeom J, Lee WH, Seo HG, Oh BM, Han TR. Characteristics of dysphagia in severe traumatic brain injury patients: a comparison with stroke patients. Ann Rehabil Med. 2016;40(3):432–9. https://doi.org/10.5535/arm.2016.40.3.432.

Leslie P, Crawford H, Wilkinson H. People with a learning disability and dysphagia: a Cinderella population? Dysphagia. 2008;24(1):103–4.

Lieberman AN, Hirowirz L, Redmond P, Pachter L, Lieberman I, Leibowitz M. Dysphagia in Parkinson's disease. Am J Gastroenterol. 1980;74:157–60.

Lindgren S, Janzon L. Prevalence of swallowing complaints and clinical findings among 50–70 year old men and women in an urban population. Dysphagia. 1991;6(4):187–92.

Llabrés M, Molina-Martinez FJ, Miralles F. Dysphagia as the sole manifestation of myasthenia gravis. J Neurol Neurosurg Psychiatry. 2005;76(9):1297–300.

Madhavan A, LaGorio LA, Crary MA, Dahl WJ, Carnaby GD. Prevalence of and risk factors for dysphagia in the community dwelling elderly: a systematic review. J Nutr Health Aging. 2016;20(8):806–15. https://doi.org/10.1007/s12603-016-0712-3.

Maeshima S, Osawa A, Miyazaki Y, Seki Y, Miura C, Tazawa Y, Tanahashi N. Influence of dysphagia on short-term outcome in patients with acute stroke. Am J Phys Med Rehabil. 2011;90(4):316–20. https://doi.org/10.1097/PHM.0b013e31820b13b2.

Manabe T, Teramoto S, Tamiya N, Okochi J, Hizawa N. Risk factors for aspiration pneumonia in older adults. PLoS One. 2015;10(10):e0140060. https://doi.org/10.1371/journal.pone.0140060.

Mandell LA, Niederman MS. Aspiration pneumonia. N Engl J Med. 2019;380(7):651–63.

Mandl T, Ekberg O, Wollmer P, Manthorpe R, Jacobsson LT. Dysphagia and dysmotility of the pharynx and oesophagus in patients with primary Sjögren's syndrome. Scand J Rheumatol. 2007;36(5):394–401. https://doi.org/10.1080/03009740701607638.

Marik PE. Aspiration pneumonitis and aspiration pneumonia. N Engl J Med. 2001;344(9):665–71.

Martino R, Foley N, Bhogal S, Diamant N, Speechley M, Teasell R. Dysphagia after stroke: incidence, diagnosis, and pulmonary complications. Stroke. 2005;36(12):2756–63. https://doi.org/10.1161/01.STR.0000190056.76543.eb.

McHorney CA, Robbins J, Lomax K, Rosenbek JC, Chignell K, Kramer AE, Bricker DE. The SWAL-QOL and SWAL-CARE outcomes tool for oropharyngeal dysphagia in adults: III. Documentation of reliability and validity. Dysphagia. 2002;17(2):97–114. https://doi.org/10.1007/s00455-001-0109-1.

Miller AJ. The neuroscientific principles of swallowing and dysphagia. San Diego: Singular; 1999.

Ministry of Health. Guidelines for the prevention of choking on food in pediatric age, edition July 2017; 2017. https://www.salute.gov.it/portale/news/p3_2_1_1_1.jsp?menu=notizie&id=3001.

Ministry of Health, Labour And Welfare. Vital statistics of Japan; 2018. www.e-stat.go.jp.

Mitsuhata T, Teramoto S. Epidemiology of aspiration pneumonia. In: Teramoto S, Komiya SK, editors. Aspiration pneumonia. Singapore: Springer; 2020.

Monte FS, da Silva-Júnior FP, Braga-Neto P, Souza NE, MÂ, Sales de Bruin VM. Swallowing abnormalities and dyskinesia in Parkinson's disease. Mov Disord. 2005;20(4):457–62. https://doi.org/10.1002/mds.20342.

Mulder DW. The diagnosis and treatment of amyotrophic lateral sclerosis. Boston: Houghton Mifflin; 1980.

Murray JP. Deglutition in myasthenia gravis. Br J Radiol. 1962;35(409):43–52.

Nakagawa K, Hara K, Tohara H. Oral care: does Oral care have preventive roles in aspiration pneumonia? In: Teramoto S, Komiya SK, editors. Aspiration pneumonia. Singapore: Springer; 2020.

Nogueira D, Reis E. Swallowing disorders in nursing home residents: how can the problem be explained? Clin Interv Aging. 2013;8:221–7.

Ntoumazios SK, Voulgari PV, Potsis K, Koutis E, Tsifetaki N, Assimakopoulos DA. Esophageal involvement in scleroderma: gastroesophageal reflux, the common problem. Semin Arthritis Rheum. 2006;36(3):173–81. https://doi.org/10.1016/j.semarthrit.2006.08.002.

Oh TH, Brumfield KA, Hoskin TL, Stolp KA, Murray JA, Bassford JR. Dysphagia in inflammatory myopathy: clinical characteristics, treatment strategies, and outcome in 62 patients. Mayo Clin Proc. 2007;82(4):441–7. https://doi.org/10.4065/82.4.441.

Park YH, Han HR, Oh BM, Lee J, Park JA, Yu SJ, Chang H. Prevalence and associated factors of dysphagia in nursing home residents. Geriatr Nurs. 2013;34(3):212–7. https://doi.org/10.1016/j.gerinurse.2013.02.014.

Parker C, Power M, Hamdy S, Bowen A, Tyrrell P, Thompson DG. Awareness of dysphagia by patients following stroke predicts swallowing performance. Dysphagia. 2004;19(1):28–35. https://doi.org/10.1007/s00455-003-0032-8.

Pauloski BR, Rademaker AW, Logemann JA, Stein D, Beery Q, Newman L, Hanchett C, Tusant S, MacCracken E. Pretreatment swallowing function in patients with head and neck cancer. Head Neck. 2000;22(5):474–82. https://doi.org/10.1002/1097-0347(200008)22:5<474::aid-hed6>3.0.co;2-i.

Paulozzi LJ, Ballesteros MF, Stevens JA. Recent trends in mortality from unintentional injury in the United States. J Saf Res. 2006;37(3):277–83.

Pauw A, Dejaeger E, D'hooghe M, Carton H. Dysphagia in multiple sclerosis. Clin Neurol Neurosurg. 2002;104(4):345–51.

Plowman E, Plowman E, Tabor L, Robison R, Wymer J, et al. Delineating mechanisms of dysphagia in ALS. Amyotroph Lateral Scler Frontotemporal Degener. 2016;17(1):33.

Potulska A, Friedman A, Królicki L, Spychala A. Swallowing disorders in Parkinson's disease. Parkinsonism Relat Disord. 2003;9(6):349–53. https://doi.org/10.1016/s1353-8020(03)00045-2.

Regional Agency For Health Services—Piedmont Region. Diagnostic therapeutic care pathway for dysphagia; 2013. https://www.regione.piemonte.it/web/sites/default/files/media/documenti/2019-01/pdta_disfagia_2013.

Restivo DA, Marchese-Ragona R, Patti F. Management of swallowing disorders in multiple sclerosis. Neurol Sci. 2006;27:338–40.

Riso S., Biroli G., D'Andrea F. (2001), Artificial nutrition, in O. Schindler, G. Ruoppolo, A. Schindler, Deglutology, Omega Editions Turin.

Robbins JA, Logemann JA, Kirshner HS. Swallowing and speech production in Parkinson's disease. Ann Neurol. 1986;19(3):283–7. https://doi.org/10.1002/ana.410190310.

Rogers B, Stratton P, Msall M, Andres M, Champlain MK, Koerner P, Piazza J. Long-term morbidity and management strategies of tracheal aspiration in adults with severe developmental disabilities. Am J Ment Retard. 1994;98(4):490–8.

Ruoppolo G, Amitrano A, Cupillo BT, Pizzorni N. Oskar Schindler and the birth of deglutology in Italy. Logopedia e Comunicazione. 2021;17(1):23–38.

Schindler O. Operational manual of pathophysiology of swallowing. Turin: Omega Editions; 1990.

Siebens H, Trupe E, Siebens A, Cook F, Anshen S, Hanauer R, Oster G. Correlates and consequences of eating dependency in institutionalized elderly. J Am Geriatr Soc. 1986;34(3):192–8. https://doi.org/10.1111/j.1532-5415.1986.tb04202.x.

Silveira Guijarro LJ, Domingo García V, Montero Fernández N, Osuna del Pozo CM, Álvarez Nebreda L, Serra-Rexach JA. Disfagia orofaríngea en ancianos ingresados en una unidad de convalecencia [Oropharyngeal dysphagia in elderly inpatients in a unit of convalescence]. Nutr Hosp. 2011;26(3):501–10. Spanish. https://doi.org/10.1590/S0212-16112011000300011.

Smithard DG, O'Neill PA, England RE, Park CL, Wyatt R, Martin DF, Morris J. The natural history of dysphagia following a stroke. Dysphagia. 1997;12(4):188–93. https://doi.org/10.1007/PL00009535.
Spadola BM, Vannucchi R, Schindler O. Psychiatric dysphagia. In: De Vincentiis M, editor. The recovery of laryngeal functions following neurological, psychiatric diseases and cervical-facial surgery. Milan: Franco Angeli; 2016a. p. 105–12.
Spadola BM, Vannucchi R, Schindler O. Psychiatric dysphagia: a proposal for nosological framing. I CARE. 2016b;41(1):16–21.
Sung HY, Kim JS, Lee KS, Kim YI, Song IU, Chung SW, Yang DW, Cho YK, Park JM, Lee IS, Kim SW, Chung IS, Choi MG. The prevalence and patterns of pharyngoesophageal dysmotility in patients with early stage Parkinson's disease. Mov Disord. 2010;25(14):2361–8. https://doi.org/10.1002/mds.23290.
Suttrup I, Warnecke T. Dysphagia in Parkinson's disease. Dysphagia. 2016;31(1):24–32.
Taniguchi Y, Iwagami M, Sakata N, Watanabe T, Abe K, Tamiya N. Epidemiology of food choking deaths in Japan: time trends and regional variations. J Epidemiol. 2021;31(5):356–60. https://doi.org/10.2188/jea.JE20200057.
Tanner DC. Case studies in communicative sciences and disorders. Columbus: Pearson Prentice Hall; 2006.
Teramoto S, Komiya K, editors. Aspiration pneumonia. Singapore: Springer; 2020.
Teramoto S, Kawashima M, Komiya K, Shoji S. Health-care-associated pneumonia is primarily due to aspiration pneumonia. Chest. 2009;136(6):1702–3. https://doi.org/10.1378/chest.09-1204.
Teramoto S, Yoshida K, Hizawa N. Update on the pathogenesis and management of pneumonia in the elderly roles of aspiration pneumonia. Respir Investig. 2015;53(5):178–84.
Thomas CL, editor. Taber's cyclopedic medical dictionary. Philadelphia: F. A. Davis; 1993.
United Nations. World population prospects 2019; 2019. https://population.un.org/wpp/.
United Nations. World population ageing 2020 highlights October 2020; 2020. https://www.un.org/development/desa/pd/.
Verdonschot RJ, Baijens L, Vanbelle S, Florie M, Kremer B, Leue C. The relationship between fiberoptic endoscopic evaluation of swallowing outcome and symptoms of anxiety and depression in dysphagic patients. Laryngoscope. 2016;126(5):E199–207. https://doi.org/10.1002/lary.25698.
Wakabayashi H. Presbyphagia and sarcopenic dysphagia: association between ageing, sarcopenia, and deglutition disorders. J Frailty Aging. 2014;3(2):97–103.
WHO (World Health Organization). Global burden of stroke 2014; 2014a. http://www.who.int/cardiovascular_diseases/en/cvd_adas_15_burden_stroke.pdf?ua=1.
WHO (World Health Organization). The top 10 causes of death, Fact Sheet n. 310; 2014b. https://www.who.int/news-room/fact-sheets/detail/the-top-10-causes-of-death.
Winstein CJ. Neurogenic dysphagia: frequency, progression and outcome in adults following brain injury. Phys Ther. 1983;63(12):1992–7.
Yorkstone KM, Honsinger MJ, Mitsuda PM, Hammen V. The relationship between speech and swallowing disorders in head-injured patients. J Head Trauma Rehabil. 1989;4(4):1–16.
Zeng R, Schmidt J. Impact and management of dysphagia in inflammatory myopathies. Curr Rheumatol Rep. 2020;22(10):74.

3 Assessment of Dysphagia in Adult Dysphagic Patients

The evaluation is the first essential moment in the care of patients with dysphagia (Logemann 1983). It can be carried out with clinical or instrumental methods, often both (McCullough and Martino 2013). It is important to formulate a diagnosis and identify the dysfunction that generates the swallowing disorder. In fact, the presence and nature of the swallowing problem are established through evaluation. In other words, an assessment is important not only for diagnostic purposes but also for stating and defining the rehabilitation program. The evaluation of dysphagia can be divided into three levels:

1. Screening (Martino et al. 2009)
2. *Clinical swallow examination* (CSE) (Carnaby-Mann and Lenius 2008; Oh et al. 2016; Leder and Espinosa 2002)
3. Instrumental evaluation (Leder and Espinosa 2002; Birchall et al. 2020).

Each level of evaluation defines, in an increasingly accurate way, the nature and degree of swallowing dysfunction.

The purpose of screening is to highlight any risk situations requiring further clinical investigation.

The second level corresponds to the *bedside examination*, which is now more correctly defined as the *clinical swallow examination (CSE)*, and consists of non-instrumental clinical evaluation: this type of evaluation is not necessarily administered to bedridden patients and aims for various and articulated purposes; it serves the following purposes:

- Detect the presence of dysphagia
- Assess its severity
- Identify the dysfunctional mechanisms

This chapter was written by Antonio Amitrano in collaboration with Giulia Rossi, a speech-language therapist.

A. Amitrano, *Dysphagia and Nutrition*,
https://doi.org/10.1007/978-3-031-77449-2_3

- Plan the rehabilitation
- Remodel a treatment plan
- Evaluate the treatment outcomes
- Initiate a therapeutic relationship

The third level of evaluation has the same objectives as the instrumental evaluation with the addition of the formulation of the diagnosis.

Each level of evaluation enriches the knowledge of patients' swallowing disorders and involves different health professionals. The screening is generally administered by a specially trained nurse. This is because the number and 24-hour presence of a nurse in the health facility better respond to the need to administer the screening to a large population, consisting of subjects over 75 years old, with neurological or respiratory diseases. The second level, or non-instrumental clinical evaluation, uses the speech therapist as the reference figure. The third level, *instrumental evaluation*, in Italy generally includes the phoniatrician, the radiologist, and the otolaryngologist (Table 3.1) as reference figures.

Table 3.1 Diagnostic tests

Diagnostic tests	Implementation methods	Advantages	Disadvantages
Screening	The patient is asked to take generally liquid medications	Rapid administration and use of easily available tools	Not reliable in cases of absence of cough reflex
Clinical non-instrumental evaluation	Medical history Analysis of swallowing organs Feeding tests	Noninvasive Use of easily available tools	Not very reliable in the absence of cough reflex Depends on the operator
Videofluoroscopy (VFS)	Swallowing radiopaque boluses of different texture	Visualization of aspirations Analysis of the entire swallowing act including the esophageal phase	Radiation exposure Transfer of the patient to the radiological environment Instrument-dependent
Fiberoptic/flexible endoscopic evaluation of swallowing (FEES)	A small endoscope inserted through the nose allows the live visualization of swallowing acts	Can be done at the bedside of the patient Direct visualization of pharynx and larynx Allows to assess the sensitivity	Invasive technique Instrument-dependent
Manometry	A small sensor inserted in the pharynx and in the esophagus measures the pressures during the swallowing act	Assessment of muscle function	Invasive technique Instrument-dependent Difficult accessibility
Scintigraphy	Swallowing of radiolabeled boluses	Visualization and quantification of aspirations	Poor anatomical definition Instrument-dependent Difficult accessibility

3.1 Clinical Evaluation

The clinical evaluation includes two different steps:

1. Screening
2. CSE

The evaluation process usually begins with the administration of screening and, for patients positive for screening tests, continues with non-instrumental clinical evaluation and subsequently with instrumental evaluation. The clinical evaluation includes a series of tests aimed at better determination of the patient's swallowing difficulties, to prepare appropriate diagnostic, care, and rehabilitation pathways. In carrying out the clinical evaluation, we observe two types of behaviors:

1. Spontaneous
2. Induced

Spontaneous *behaviors* are those that the evaluator can detect in the early stages of the encounter, when the narration of the swallowing disorder is collected directly from the patient where possible. Several types of *spontaneous behavior* are observed: the first of which is vocal quality. In fact, some types of voice, such as the "wet voice," are indicators of aspiration and therefore represent a strong indication of the presence of dysphagia. Verbal production is also observed because often, in patients with dysphagia, there is a coexisting dysarthric disorder, the characterization of which can provide useful hints to the clinician to define the patient's swallowing dysfunction. The possible presence of facial asymmetries indicating the involvement of the seventh cranial facial nerve should be noted and may presage the presence of bolus residues within the plegic cheek after the oral phase. At the first meeting with patients, it is also important to detect how they manage their saliva. There may be drooling, or patients may spit out the saliva they cannot swallow. These behaviors are both signs of swallowing problems, albeit different ones. In the following step of the evaluation, *induced behaviors* are evaluated, i.e., the patient is asked to perform some specific actions. In this case, the possible presence of buccofacial apraxia (BFA), a disorder of voluntary and imitative motor skills, must be carefully investigated. Buccofacial apraxia limits the patient's ability to perform voluntary movements but does not hinder the execution of automatic or involuntary movements. Its presence negatively affects the patient's performance on tests investigating oral motor functionality but not necessarily during swallowing in everyday life situations because, in this case, mainly automatic and reflex movements are used. At this stage of the evaluation, patients are asked to perform specific movements with the organs involved in the execution of the swallowing act. Each of them is evaluated in the execution of movements according to its own directions of movement: for example, the tongue is asked for movements of protrusion, retraction, lateralization, and lifting. The analysis of the motor behavior of the swallowing organs is followed by feeding tests, during which the patient is asked to swallow boluses of different volumes and textures. This is certainly the most delicate and risky phase of the evaluation and should be performed only when patients are alert and able to control a sitting position. The feeding tests are not performed in cases of severe impairment of oral motor skills. Feeding tests must be performed following adequate oral hygiene.

3.1.1 Dysphagia Screening

Screening is a simple and quick method that aims not only to diagnose dysphagia but also to detect potential risk situations that require further and more detailed evaluation procedures. In other words, after administering a screening test, it is not possible to affirm that the patient has dysphagia but only that they are at risk of dysphagia. In these cases, the patient must be directed toward a more accurate evaluation process, carried out by operators with a greater degree of specific skills. Screening tests are necessarily simple, as they present, in their ease and speed of administration, an important criterion of applicability. It is indeed unlikely that an operator, which is generally burdened with multiple tasks, can have adequate time to use sensitive and precise scales, moreover requiring long administration times. Dysphagia screening is a set of simple methodologies whose main references are represented by the signs of dysphagia. The important characteristics of screening are *sensitivity*, which is the ability to identify true positives, which must range between 80% and 90%, and *specificity*, which is the ability to identify true negatives, which should be at least 50%. The feasibility of a screening program is linked to the presence of certain requirements:

- *Epidemiological requirements*: the disease must have a sufficient prevalence in the population.
- *Diagnostic requirements*: tests must be easily administered to a large population.
- *Therapeutic requirements*: the possibility of using therapies that can slow down or nullify the consequences of the disease.
- *Prognostic requirements*: advantages in the social and working life of the subject whose disease has been diagnosed earlier.
- *Economic requirements*: the screening must reduce the social cost caused by the disease, owing to the better performance achievable with rehabilitation.

Dysphagia is a very common problem in at-risk populations, with significant prevalence rates in the general population, especially in elderly individuals, as already observed in CAP. 2. The second requirement for the feasibility of a screening program is linked to the existence of easily applicable screening tools in a large population. To date, numerous screening tests have been reported in the literature: the tools proposed by various authors have different characteristics, and many of them have good psychometric characteristics of validity and reliability. The number of available tests allows the clinician to identify the most suitable tool to apply to specific realities. The third requirement for the feasibility of a screening program is related to the availability of specific therapies that can slow down or nullify the consequences of the disease—in our case, dysphagia. Rehabilitation will be discussed more extensively in CAP. 4, while there are currently numerous techniques available to the rehabilitator, allowing an intervention in patients with various swallowing dysfunctions. In general, rehabilitative treatment is based on two distinct strategies: *direct intervention for symptoms* and *compensation*. Both strategies, with different methods and techniques, attempt to restore a safe and adequate per os feeding from a nutritional point of view. With respect to the prognostic and economic requirements, screening for dysphagia reduces the risk of complications such as pneumonia *ab ingestis*, dependence on feeding tubes, and death. Dysphagia seriously endangers the survival of the subject, both for the risk of choking and for the possibility of passing through part of the bolus into the lower airways, with the possible occurrence of aspiration pneumonia, whose risk is tripled compared with that of patients without swallowing alterations (Martino et al. 2005). The onset of aspiration pneumonia is associated with a tripled risk of mortality for dysphagic patients (Katzan et al. 2003). Dysphagia also causes malnutrition and dehydration (Foley et al. 2009) and makes the use of oral therapy problematic. Early evaluation of dysphagia has significant impacts on health, hospitalization times, and, ultimately, patient health costs (Foley et al. 2009; Donovan et al. 2013). Consequently, dysphagia screening fully meets the criteria required for the implementation of a screening program. Moreover, the need to subject patients to a screening procedure before resuming feeding per os is an indication given by numerous guidelines. The most commonly used screening test, which is included in all screening cards, is the *water glass test*, which consists of asking the patient, who is alert and able to maintain the sitting position, to independently drink a glass of water in a quiet environment. The presence of cough or the modification of vocal quality after bolus intake makes the test result positive and decreases the referral of the patient to subsequent levels of evaluation. The test should be suspended as soon as the patient coughs. The water glass test was proposed by De Pippo et al. (1992), who asked the patient to drink at his own pace 3 oz., equivalent to approximately 85 ml, of water. The test is positive; that is, it provides evidence of swallowing dysfunction, if cough or a wet voice occurs while the patient is drinking or within a minute from the end of the test. The test can be performed if the patient is alert and can maintain the sitting position upright and must be performed in a quiet environment. Different methods of administering water glass tests have subsequently been proposed, which introduce a criterion of graduality in the administration of water boluses. Initially, 5 ml of smooth water was added at room temperature with a teaspoon three times, to ensure that the patient had swallowed. If the patient has a cough and/or a gurgling voice, the test is suspended; if there are no problems, 85 ml of water is drawn directly from the glass, and then the patient is asked to speak to verify any modification in vocal quality. The author reported a sensitivity of 80% and a specificity of 54% for the water glass test. Patients who test positive in the screening are cautiously put on a feeding pause until the outcome of the subsequent evaluation levels is reached. This element places the sequence of evaluation levels in a precise temporal order that does not allow long intervals between one level and the other. The water glass test, like all clinical tests, may be less sensitive because of the possible absence of the cough reflex. In these cases, the examiner has no evidence on which to base the suspicion of bolus passage into the airways. To increase the sensitivity of the water glass test, combining it with cervical auscultation and simultaneous measurement of oxygen saturation with a pulse oximeter have been proposed. *Pulse oximetry* is a method for detecting the level of oxygen saturation in the blood and is used for the evaluation of the oxygenation status of patients, with the application of a probe in an area pervaded by surface circulation. The technique is based on the fact that the inhaled bolus stimulates laryngeal chemoreceptors, causing reflex bronchoconstriction, altering ventilation, and producing desaturation of arterial blood oxygen. However, today, the main guidelines indicate pulse oximetry as a test that provides additional information to the clinical evaluation of dysphagia, but that cannot be considered the only way to determine the presence of dysphagia (Firino and Raimondo 2019). *Cervical auscultation* is based on the use of a stethoscope, a microphone, or an accelerometer placed on the surface of the front part of the neck, in contact with the skin near the larynx. In this way, the sounds and vibrations that are generated during swallowing (Leslie et al. 2004) are detected. This method is used to collect information on the pharyngeal phase, the coordination between breathing and swallowing, and the possible penetration or aspiration into the upper airways. In the case of swallowing dysfunctions, alterations in the acoustic signal are detected (Logemann et al. 1999). Auscultation is recognized as a valid technique, but, if used in isolation, it does not allow the identification of all episodes of oropharyngeal aspiration (Firino and Raimondo 2019).

Numerous tests have been proposed for dysphagia screening: among these tests, the *Toronto Bedside Swallowing Screening Test* (TOR-BSST) (Martino et al. 2009) has been validated in a population of patients with stroke. The test can be administered by specially trained healthcare personnel, for whom a training course is required, which the authors have quantified in 4 h. The test is simple to perform and can be used both in acute hospitals and in rehabilitation. The TOR-BSST has a sensitivity of 91.3% and analyzes three different behaviors:

1. Ability to swallow liquid boluses
2. Tongue strength
3. Voice before and after the swallowing test

The test is divided into two parts that require approximately 10 min for administration:

1. The first part explains the importance of the evaluation and indicates useful tools to determine the presence of dysphagia (physical examination and swallowing ability) and contains two items that analyze voice and lingual motility.
2. The second part includes swallowing ability tests and the detection of consequent behaviors.

As with other screening tests, for it to be administered, the patient must be alert and must sit with the back of the bed raised to 90°. In the first part of the test, the patient is asked to pronounce the vowel "a" and then to stick out their tongue. If the voice is normal, presenting no type of anomalies, and if the tongue in the protrusion does not deviate, we move on to the second part. In the second part, the patient is asked to sequentially drink ten teaspoons full of water. With each spoon administered, it is checked if there is a cough or modification of the voice: the test is suspended if one of the two phenomena occurs. In this case, in fact, the test receives the outcome "fail," and the patient is put on a nil per os regimen and referred to speech therapy evaluation. If, on the other hand, the ten teaspoons are taken without any manifestation of pathological behaviors, the patient is asked to drink a glass of water and then to produce the vowel "A." Similarly, in this case, if the voice does not change and there is no cough, the test receives the outcome "pass." Subject to copyright, the TOR-BSST can be administered only by certified personnel.

The *volume-viscosity test* (VVST) (Clavé et al. 2008) is a clinical test used to identify signs of swallowing alteration, with a sensitivity of 88% and a specificity of 64%. The test was validated through a sample of 97 subjects whose test performances were compared with performances in a task similar to the videofluoroscopic examination. To increase the sensitivity of the test, saturation was measured with a pulse oximeter during administration. The test involves the evaluation of swallowing performance during the ingestion of boluses of varying volume and consistency. The consistencies tested are liquid, nectar, and pudding. The presentation volumes of the various consistencies are 5, 10, and 20 ml.

The following were considered signs of poor swallowing safety:

- Cough
- Decrease in saturation ≥3%
- Changes in voice quality

The following were considered signs of alterations in swallowing efficiency:

- Fractionated swallowing
- Presence of residues in the oral cavity and pharynx

The administration of the test requires the availability of the following materials:

- Water
- Thickener in prepackaged sachets of 4.5 g and 9 g
- A glass
- A 20 ml syringe
- A spoon
- A pulse oximeter

The test was carried out with the pulse oximeter positioned on the index finger of the right hand. The baseline value against which to detect any desaturations is detected 2 min before the start of the test. The administration of the boluses continues from the smallest volume to the largest volume. Textures are administered according to the sequence of nectar, liquid, and pudding. A flow chart of the methods used to administer the test under various possible clinical conditions is available to the examiner. The duration of the administration is, according to the authors' indications, less than 6 min. The criteria for access to screening are as follows:

- Patients over 75 years old
- Patients with respiratory diseases
- Patients with neurological diseases

The *Royal Brisbane and Woman Hospital* (RBWH) dysphagia screening tool (Cichero et al. 2009) is a screening test for dysphagia that, unlike the vast majority of validated screening tests with stroke patient populations, has been validated on a population of patients in a general acute care hospital. RBWH is a nursing tool, as screening tests are generally performed and are applicable to heterogeneous patient populations in acute care units. The test has been translated and validated for use in the Italian context in a sample of 105 patients (Mozzanica et al. 2017). It requires a short specific training course, quantified by the authors as approximately 30 min, has a sensitivity of 95% and a specificity of 97%, and is divided into two phases, the second of which is further divided into three steps. The total administration time is approximately 9 min, of which approximately 2 min are needed for the first phase and approximately 5–7 min for the second. In the first phase, the presence of conditions commonly associated with dysphagia is detected: if the patient does not present any of the clinical conditions commonly associated with dysphagia, the nurse stops the screening, and the patient is fed a normal diet. If instead the patient presents one of the clinical conditions commonly associated with dysphagia, the second phase of the test is conducted; the first step involves interviewing the patient or family members, and the second step involves detecting the presence of dysphagia or signs of aspiration. If the patient does not show any signs of dysphagia, the water glass test included in the third step of the test is performed. Otherwise, in the event that the patient shows signs of dysphagia, the nurse stops the screening, puts the patient on a nil per os regimen, and refers them to the speech therapist for further evaluation.

The *Gugging Swallowing Screen* (GUSS) (Trapl et al. 2007) is another screening tool validated through a validation process carried out in comparison with the *Fiberoptic Endoscopic Evaluation of Swallowing* (FEES) in 50 patients with acute stroke. The test is divided into two parts: the first part includes indirect swallowing tests; the second part includes three subtests that analyze the patient's ability to swallow three different textures offered in a specific order. The different parts of the test must be administered sequentially. Each item provides for the assignment of a score to the performance carried out by the patient. The highest score is assigned to the best performance, whereas the lowest score is assigned to the worst performance. The maximum score of the test is 20, with each of the four subtests having a maximum score of 5. The test is administered with the patient seated and in a quiet environment. The textures and devices used during the test must be presented in a frontal position. The first section assesses the prerequisites necessary for the performance of subsequent feeding tests. If the patient achieves an adequate score on the vigilance test (presence of cough and swallowing of saliva), the second section is as follows: a score of 5 in the first section allows progression to the second; otherwise, the test is suspended, the patient is put on *nothing by mouth*, and a subsequent evaluation is scheduled. The second section includes feeding tests that are first performed for semisolids (jellified water), then for liquids (water), and finally for solids (dry bread). If each of the three tests is passed without signs of dysfunction, i.e., without cough, voice changes, and drooling, the following texture is processed. The test is stopped at any point where coughing or another dysfunctional phenomenon occurs. Depending on the scores obtained on the test, a diet for the patient's feeding can be identified. A score of 20 suggests a normal diet, without restrictions, and a score of 15–19 suggests an adapted diet devoid of solid foods. A score of 10–14 suggests a creamy diet that does not include liquids. A score of 0–9 does not allow any oral feeding.

For the identification of dysphagia in patients in the intensive care unit—(ICU), a version of the GUSS, the GUSS-ICU, has recently been proposed (Troll et al. 2023). The GUSS-ICU applies to a specific population and includes the Richmond Agitation-Sedation Scale (RASS) (Sessler et al. 2002), a scale that assesses patients' degree of agitation. The GUSS-ICU employs the IDDSI framework to determine the needed food textures.

The *Dysphagia Risk Score 2* (DRS2) (Amitrano et al. 2023) is another screening tool. The DRS2 was validated by comparing it with FEES. The study involved 1006 patients (499 females and 507 males), aged between 15 and 101 years (with an average of 70 years), evaluated with the DRS2 within 24–48 h of admission. For the purpose of validating the scale, among the 1006 patients, a random sample of 169 subjects (100 males and 69 females, average age 71 years) was also subjected to an examination with FEES during the same diagnostic session. The DRS2 is the updated version of the *Dysphagia Risk Score* (DRS), proposed by Amitrano and Pezzella (2009). The DRS is a scale model that aims to calculate the risk of the onset of dysphagia complications: it is a hierarchical scale that involves the execution of simple tests that are part of the practice of *nursing*. The scale consists of nine items: patient's age, level of consciousness, ability to execute simple orders, water test, cough test, presence or absence of wet voice, presence of drooling, patient's ability to actively eliminate saliva, and presence of dyspnea. In light of the experience accumulated over the years of experimental use of the DRS, the authors have proposed the second version of the DRS, which, unlike the first version, has undergone a complete validation process. *Dysphagia Risk Score 2* comes from the simplification of the items of the first version, with a further reduction in administration times. The DRS2, in fact, consists of eight items presented in a different order than the first version.

The eight items that make up the scale are as follows:

1. *Patient's age*: A score of 1 is assigned to subjects who have reached or exceeded 75 years of age.

2. *Level of consciousness*: In the absence of vigilance, a score of 1 is assigned, and the administration of the scale is interrupted, assigning the patient the maximum risk value.
3. *Voluntary cough*: The patient's inability to cough on verbal request or imitation results in a score of 3.
4. *Water test*: The patient was asked to drink approximately 90 cc of water. If coughing occurred during the test or within a minute of administering the water, a score of 3 was assigned. The test is stopped if the patient starts to cough.
5. *Voice quality*: In the presence of a change in voice quality after administering the glass of water, a score of 3 is assigned.
6. *Presence of drooling*: A score of 0.5 is assigned.
7. *Saliva emission*: If during the entire observation the patient autonomously spits saliva, this behavior is assigned a score of 3.
8. *Dyspnea*: In the case of clear breathing difficulty, a score of 2 is assigned.

All the scores obtained, excluding 0, activate further procedures for evaluating swallowing and result in the precautionary suspension of oral feeding. In other words, the screening is passed ("pass") with a score of 0 and failed ("fail") in all other cases.

3.1.2 Clinical Swallow Examination

Patients who test positive in the screening require a further level of evaluation, which is more accurate and is administered by staff with a greater degree of specific preparation for swallowing disorders. The next level after screening is the bedside examination, a term once widely used and progressively replaced by the more correct clinical swallowing examination (CSE) or non-instrumental clinical evaluation. This definition, in fact, better describes the operation of a type of evaluation that is applicable to all patient conditions and is not restricted to bedridden patients, as the old definition might erroneously suggest. In Italy the non-instrumental clinical evaluation is carried out by the speech-language therapist and aims to confirm the suspicion of dysphagia that emerged during the screening and, when possible, to identify the dysfunctional mechanisms that generate dysphagia. The non-instrumental clinical evaluation consists of three different phases: the first is composed of the collection of the patient's medical history, the second is from the morphodynamic analysis of the structures and organs involved in swallowing, and the third is from feeding tests. In the first phase of the evaluation, when possible, the information that the patient provides about the timing and methods of onset of the swallowing disorder, as well as the subjective localization of symptoms, is collected. These elements guide the subsequent analysis of the individual organs involved in swallowing. The complexity of the investigation increases as we move from the most external anatomical structures, which are therefore more visible and better explorable, toward the inside. It is relatively easy to observe the motility of the lips and tongue, while it is slightly more complex to observe the motility of the palatine veil, and it is impossible, with a clinical methodology, to observe pharyngeal and laryngeal motility. When performing CSE for the analysis of the inner structures of the swallowing tract, the evaluator must draw appropriate inferences. In particular, for the functionality of the larynx analysis, the acoustic evaluation of the quality of the voice will be important. Voice variations, in fact, can indicate various laryngeal dysfunctions. If, in the screening phase, the evaluator is asked exclusively to report the modification of the voice after the intake of the liquid bolus, in the CSE, a careful perceptual analysis of vocal parameters can highlight various dysfunctions. A nasal sound indicates a possible impairment in the functionality of the palatine veil. A voice with a high degree of dysphonia may indicate a deficit in the closure of the glottic plane, whereas a wet voice generally indicates the penetration of saliva into the larynx. Additionally, the analysis of pharyngeal functionality is largely carried out by resorting to inferences. The presence of post-swallowing cough or the sensation reported by the patient of a foreign body sensation in the throat can reveal pharyngeal dysfunction. The observation of the motility of the pharyngolaryngeal tract requires instrumental techniques of analysis. In the third phase of CSE, feeding tests are administered. This is the riskiest phase, as the patient is exposed to the possibility of aspiration; for this reason, the feeding tests are always administered after the examination of the swallowing organs, and foods are proposed in a predetermined sequence: liquids, semisolids, semiliquids, and solids. In this sequence, solid foods, when possible, are tested last, as they expose the patient to the risk of choking. Not necessarily all consistencies are tested. When coughing occurs after the ingestion of liquids, the administration of semiliquid and semisolid foods proceeds. If coughing occurs with these consistencies, the test is interrupted, and solid foods are not tested. The presence of this reflex is of fundamental importance, because it allows the examiner to infer the presence of a *false route*. In fact, when evaluating patients who do not have a cough reflex, the examiner has no elements to identify a *false route*. While the instrumental evaluation allows visualization of the passage of the bolus into the airways, in the CSE, detecting the presence of cough is of fundamental importance to suspect the passage of the bolus into the lower airways. Moreover, the determination of the *timing* of the cough also allows us to hypothesize the site of the functional damage. The *three-finger test* allows not only the detection of the presence of cough but also the establishment of the phase in which the oropharyngeal transit of the bolus arises (Fig. 3.1). The examiner uses three fingers of his own hand: the index finger, the middle finger, and the ring finger. The index finger is positioned under the patient's chin (1), while the middle and ring fingers are positioned on the neck. The middle finger is positioned on the upper edge of the thyroid cartilage (2), and the ring finger is positioned on the lower edge of the cricoid cartilage (3). The patient is administered boluses of the tested consistency.

In the oral preparation phase, the examiner, with his or her index finger, perceives the movements of the tongue, whereas with the middle and ring fingers, he or she does not feel any movement. A possible cough that occurs in this phase is defined as a pre-swallowing fall. In the next phase, which roughly corresponds to the pharyngeal phase, the examiner detects, with the middle and ring fingers, the

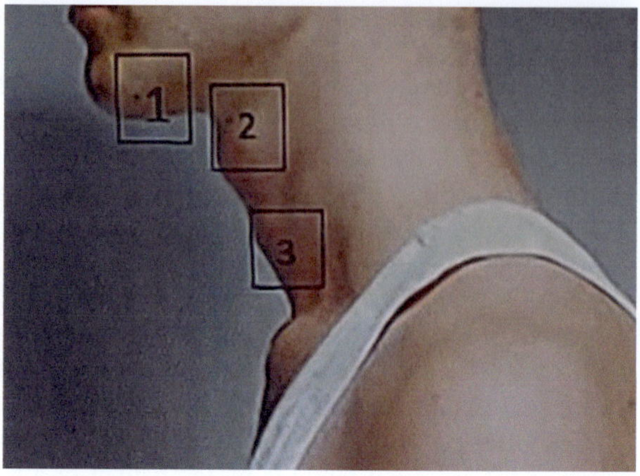

Fig. 3.1 The three-finger test

vertical excursion of the larynx. If a cough arises in this phase, it is referred to as an intra-swallowing fall. In the next phase, which corresponds to the return of the larynx to its respiratory position and at the beginning of the esophageal phase, the examiner will not feel any movement under his fingers. When a cough arises in this phase, it is referred to as a post-swallowing fall. Establishing the exact moment of cough onset helps the examiner better understand dysfunction during the course of swallowing. In fact, a pre-swallowing fall directs the search for dysfunction in the oral phase and/or the transition from the oral to the pharyngeal phase. If, in the acoustic analysis of the voice, the presence of a nasal sound is detected, swallowing dysfunction is likely to be sought in the hypofunctionality of the palatine veil. The intra-swallowing fall, on the other hand, points toward a deficit of glottic or laryngeal continence in general, which will then be confirmed or not confirmed by subsequent instrumental investigations that allow the functionality of the larynx to be visualized. A post-swallowing cough, ultimately accompanied by the sensation of a foreign body reported by the patient, drives the examiner toward the hypothesis of a disorder affecting the pharyngeal phase. The three-finger test, therefore, while not replacing the necessary instrumental investigations, allows the examiner to better clarify swallowing dysfunction. Moreover, during the implementation of the rehabilitation program, the three-finger test provides continuous feedback to the speech therapist and the patient himself. All forms of non-instrumental evaluation have an insurmountable Achilles heel in the absence of the cough reflex (Battel et al. 2016). Non-instrumental clinical evaluation is based on the administration of specific protocols. Many tools are available in the literature, two of which have been validated, such as the *Mann Assessment of Swallowing Ability* (MASA) (Mann 2002; Kwon et al. 2019) and the *Functional Oral Intake Scale* (FOIS) (Crary et al. 2005; Battel et al. 2018), and others that, although in use in clinical practice, have not been subjected to validation processes.

One of these is the dysphagia assessment protocol developed by speech therapist Francoise Cot and occupational therapist Guylaine Desharnais (Cot and Desharnais 1985). This protocol has the advantage of presenting itself as a complete checklist of the different aspects that need to be observed in the evaluation of dysphagic patients. The first part of the test collects the main demographic and anamnestic information related to the patient, followed by the data on his current feeding methods and the state of his breathing. Information on the symptoms reported by the patient is also noted, particularly whether or not he or she reports episodes in a *false way*, on the level of communication, on eating habits, and on the presence of any food allergies or intolerances. In the next section, the morphology and motility of the various swallowing organs are analyzed. The analysis of head movements is not conducted for diagnostic purposes, but is a useful element for the programming of the rehabilitative intervention. In fact, one of the tools of rehabilitation is postural compensation, which is adopted to modify the flow of the bolus in the swallowing channel. For the rehabilitator, it is therefore useful to know the patient's ability to perform the neck movements necessary for the use of postural compensation maneuvers. The superficial, deep, thermal, and taste sensitivities of the various parts of the mouth and face are also investigated. The presence of normal reflexes (cough reflex, vomiting, and swallowing) and pathological reflexes (bite and suction reflex) was analyzed. At the end of the test, the feeding tests are performed, which constitute the riskiest part of the test and must be administered when the patient has a good level of alertness and sufficient oral movements. In other words, the feeding tests should not be administered in cases where the patient is not alert and oral motility is absent. In the last part of the protocol, how the patient manages saliva, if there is drooling, and if he spits saliva or swallows it regularly are analyzed. It is important to check the state of the dentition, i.e., whether the patient is edentulous or wears dental prostheses. We also investigated whether a cough does not result from the ingestion of food or the quality of the voice. The last item analyzes whether the patient can maintain the sitting position.

The *Mann Assessment of Swallowing Ability* (MASA) (Mann 2002) is the first clinical dysphagia assessment test with good psychometric characteristics and was developed by Mann (2002) as a tool for identifying swallowing disorders in stroke patients. The test consists of 24 items that investigate 4 main areas:

- General patient status
- Oral preparation phase
- Oral phase
- Pharyngeal phase

Each area is in turn composed of several items.

- General patient status (8 items):
  - Responsiveness
  - Cooperation
  - Auditory comprehension
  - Breathing
  - Breathing-swallowing coordination

  - Aphasia
  - Apraxia
  - Dysarthria
- Oral preparation (6 items):
  - Saliva
  - Lip continence
  - Tongue motility
  - Tongue strength
  - Tongue coordination
  - Oral preparation
- Oral phase (4 items):
  - Gag reflex
  - Palate
  - Bolus management
  - Oral transit
- Pharyngeal phase (6 items):
  - Cough reflex
  - Voluntary cough
  - Voice
  - Tracheal cannula
  - The pharyngeal phase of swallowing
  - Pharyngeal response

Each item is assigned a maximum score of 5 or 10 points. The worst performances receive a lower score, depending on the extent of the impairment. The maximum score obtainable on the test is 200.

The cutoff is 177 for dysphagia and 170 for the risk of aspiration. Depending on the score obtained on the test, the examiner will be able to classify dysphagia as (Table 3.2):

- Absent
- Mild
- Moderate
- Severe

The score obtained allows the classification of the risk of aspiration, which is as follows (Table 3.3):

- Absent

Table 3.2 Severity of dysphagia on the basis of MASA scores

Dysphagia	MASA score
Absent	≥178
Moderate	168–177
Severe	≤138

Table 3.3 Risk of aspiration on the basis of MASA scores

Aspiration risk	MASA score
Absent	≥170
Mild	149–169
Medium	141–148
Severe	≤140

- Mild
- Medium
- Severe

As a tool for predicting aspiration in stroke patients, the MASA has a sensitivity of 93% and a specificity of 55%. As a tool for predicting dysphagia in stroke patients, however, it has a sensitivity of 71% and a specificity of 72%. The clinical evaluation tests also include diet level scales. These tools describe the patient's current diet level and are therefore tools that provide little information on the anatomical location of swallowing dysfunction. However, they allow for the planning of the patient's diet level.

These scales prove their usefulness, particularly in the quantification of the *outcome* and in the *follow-up* of dysphagic patients. The *Functional Oral Intake Scale* (FOIS) is a valid and reliable tool for measuring a patient's diet level (Crary et al. 2005). It is a seven-level ordinal scale that describes the patient's diet level: level 1 nil per os represents the highest level of severity, whereas level 7 (completely oral feeding, without any limitation) naturally constitutes the least severe level. The intermediate levels describe different situations: levels 1–3 describe various types of tube feeding, and levels 4–7 instead define the various degrees of oral feeding. The FOIS has been translated and validated into Italian (Battel et al. 2018). Among the diet-level scales are also the *Dysphagia Outcome Severity Scale* (DOSS) (O'Neil et al. 1999), whose Italian version was curated by Professor Antonio Schindler. The DOSS also describes seven diet levels, and for each level, the corresponding diet and degree of independence are indicated, as well as the type of nutrition. Finally, for each of the seven levels, patient management guidelines are also provided. Another level scale is the *National Outcome Measurement System* (NOMS), prepared by ASHA (1998). The Italian version was curated by Professor A. Schindler, and this tool also identifies seven levels for the classification of the diet level of dysphagic patients: level 7 describes a condition of substantial normality, and level 1, on the other hand, describes the inability to feed orally. In this case, feeding takes place entirely non-orally through tubes (nasogastric tube, NGT, or percutaneous endoscopic gastrostomy, PEG).

3.2 Instrumental Evaluation

Instrumental analysis allows for a clear and unequivocal illustration of all phases of swallowing (Fattori et al. 2016). However, instrumental analysis is closely linked to the availability of tools and, as in the case of videofluoroscopy (VFS), the ability to move the patient to suitable environments, which is not always feasible, as in the case of patients admitted to intensive care units. Instrumental evaluation is a level of medical evaluation with the considerable merit of clearly and unequivocally identifying episodes of aspiration. FEES does not allow for direct visualization of aspiration, but through the analysis of residues, it allows for inference of the passage of the bolus into the lower airways. Videofluoroscopy, on the other hand, allows for the visualization of aspirations as they occur through direct visualization of the passage of the bolus. This method, however, does not allow for the quantification of the bolus that passes into the larynx, which is instead possible with scintigraphy, a technique with poor morphological definition but which allows, accompanied by others, both the detection of the passage of the bolus in the subglottic area and the quantification of ingestions. Another method, still mainly used for research purposes and rarely in routine deglutology, is manometry, which allows for the measurement of the pressure developed by the different pharyngoesophageal districts with special probes. Instrumental methods represent the gold standard of swallowing evaluation, which generally concludes with this level of analysis. Notably, the use of instrumental methods is linked to the availability of technical and human resources suitable for their use. Moreover, while they constitute an indispensable moment in the diagnostic framing of the patient's swallowing disorders, they cannot be the means of daily monitoring the patient's progress in his rehabilitative journey. It is therefore important for the rehabilitator to acquire skills and abilities in evaluating the patient's disorders, to monitor his progress daily or his possible, even if not desirable, worsening. It is also desirable that in the not too distant future in Italy, the rehabilitator, after an adequate training course, can use endoscopic tools (FEES), for the sole purpose of monitoring the progress of rehabilitation and providing the patient with feedback on his own swallowing.

3.3 Mealtime Observation

In recent years, several authors have proposed an additional level of evaluation: mealtime observation (Amitrano and Crinelli 2005). Meal observation does not replace previous evaluation methods but integrates them, considering that swallowing is a dynamic fact that takes a variable amount of time and occurs in a specific context. During clinical feeding trials, the boluses of different consistencies that the patient must take are a few, and most importantly, the test itself takes place in a setting that is different from the usual setting in which the subject takes meals. In fact, the tests normally in use are based on the intake of small amounts of boluses of different consistencies (Logemann 1983), and during instrumental tests, the patient, in unnatural positions, often takes boluses of unfamiliar taste (Lambert et al. 2003). In mealtime observation, on the other hand, the behavior analysis applies to the entire duration of the meal, which is in no way conditioned by the examiner. Another distinctive element of mealtime observation is that, unlike other clinical evaluation tests, the examiner observes the patient incognito in a moment of his or her daily life to exclude or, more realistically, reduce the conditioning that the observer has on the performance of the observed patient (Gatti 2002). Observing what actually takes place while the patient is consuming meals is helpful in achieving the difficult goal of arriving at a correct definition of the swallowing disorder, since the ultimate purpose of the evaluative process is to provide the most likely evidence of swallowing performance (Lambert et al. 2003).

The purpose of mealtime observation is to gather information on how the subject with dysphagia, or suspected dysphagia, actually consumes meals in his own environment, which can be the hospital for inpatients or his own home for outpatients (ibid.). The need to create a tool for analysing a behavioral sample different from the one obtained during the assessment arises from the empirical evidence of the discrepancy in behaviors that can be noted in subjects observed in a therapeutic setting rather than in natural contexts. Patients who, for example, do not reveal coughing during the intake of liquids in an evaluative setting, quite randomly, in natural situations such as a normal consumption at the bar without any external control, showed instead coughing. Mealtime observation, in addition to being a method of completing the patient's diagnostic process, is a way to analyse and verify the setting in which the patient actually consumes his or her meal. Very often, the conditions under which a subject consumes his meals can differ in several aspects from those observed during the specific therapy session for swallowing. With respect to mealtime observation, how much the patient follows the given instructions and how much the setting is suitable for meal consumption in protected conditions are analyzed. It is quite evident that this method applies to medium-mild patients or those improving, for whom meal consumption is planned, although with limitations concerning the consistency of food or instructions regarding the required postures. Patients have a low degree of *compliance* or conformity to the therapist's instructions (Rosenvinge and Starke 2005). Often, television can either be a source of distraction or encourage incorrect postures during a meal. Generally placed in high positions in hospital rooms, television forces patients who are used to watching television programs during mealtime to a posture of head extension, possibly contrary to the given instructions and, in any case, increasing the incidence of *aspiration*. This element may not emerge in a formal evaluation, but this does not reduce its importance for framing the disorder and for safe meal consumption. Mealtime observation is carried out *blindly* which constitutes a strength of the method and, at the same time, a weak point due to the difficulty of hiding the observer in the environment where the subject usually consumes meals. Almost all the tools involve the caregiver, who, more easily than an external evaluator, can disguise the objective. The presence of the speech therapist during mealtime most likely induces the subject to use the compensation adopted in therapy. When the collaboration of the caregiver is not possible, the speech therapist will observe the subject declaring a different observation target. This condition is easily achievable in a dining room where, for example, the speech therapist declares observing a different patient from the one actually examined. Other methods, such as a one-way mirror or the use of cameras, are almost always not available in normal hospitals or domestic situations. Mealtime observation by nature requires a long time and is exclusively practicable during mealtimes. This limits its use, at least in situations where the absence of a trained caregiver makes it necessary for the therapist to administer. Moreover, timely observation allows for the analysis of swallowing problems associated with different meals. In some subjects, differentiated behaviors can be detected: usually the most problematic meals are breakfast and dinner. Breakfast is sometimes consumed in bed, with possibly inadequate postures and an uncertain state of vigilance. Dinner is the meal that ends the day and is affected by the fatigue previously accumulated. There are several tools presented for meal observation. The *Meal Observation Grid* (see *Appendix*, *Card B*) is a qualitative analysis tool for mealtime (Amitrano and Crinelli 2005) and consists of two sections: the first includes the collection of anamnestic and demographic data, and the second consists of 42 binary response items that analyze the different aspects of behaviors that occur during a meal. In the end, the examiner must indicate the total time that the subject took to consume the meal. The test does not have a score but provides the examiner with a broad and fairly exhaustive picture of the ways in which the subject consumes the meal. The examiner is the speech therapist or a specifically trained caregiver. When the *Meal Observation Grid* is used as a final verification tool for a treatment, it is appropriate that the examiner is different from the speech therapist who carried out the treatment. In this case, a conditioning would be created that would make the data acquired unreliable. The meal observation tool used is the *McGill Ingestive Skills Assessment* (MISA) (Lambert et al. 2003). This tool is also available in the Italian version of the MISA-I (Lambert 2011) and includes 43 items divided into 5 scales:

1. Positioning during meals (4 items)
2. Ability to feed oneself (7 items)
3. Oral movements for the ingestion of solid foods (12 items)
4. Oral movements for the ingestion of liquid foods (7 items)
5. Management of consistencies (13 items)

The different items are reported on a three-point ordinal scale. A score of 3 indicates the best performance, whereas a score of 1 indicates the worst performance. The score is differentiated by scale, and the sum of the scores of the five scales results in the total score. The MISA is a scale designed for the evaluation and treatment of adults and elderly individuals with neurogenic dysphagia, rather than surgical or neoplastic dysphagia. The MISA must be administered during the observation of a meal that the therapist observes sitting about 6 feet (approximately 2 metres) from the patient. The observer sits in a position that allows him to see the patient's mouth eating without being invasive. Interacting verbally with the patient is forbidden to the observer, except for minimal interactions to establish a courtesy report and actively intervene in the ways in which the patient consumes meals. If the patient is normally assisted by a caregiver, he also provides his service during the observation for the administration of the MISA. If feeding is judged harmful to the patient, it will be interrupted simultaneously with the administration of MISA.

Another tool for meal observation is the Mealtime Assessment Scale (MAS) (Valentini et al. 2015). This is a quantitative tool that allows the evaluation of a subject with suspected or confirmed dysphagia. The observation setting is that of the common meal that the subject consumes without any indication from the examiner, who has the role of an external observer. The scale consists of three different sections plus one. The first three sections have scores ranging from 0 to 3, where the highest score indicates behaviors that fall within the norm and the score 0 indicates the maximum deficit. The first section (*preliminary indications*) is dedicated to the collection of the psychophysical and cognitive characteristics of the examinee. The second section (*rheological characteristics of food and nutrition methods*) collects information on food and on the size of the bolus that the subject takes during the meal. The third section (*signs of dysphagia at mealtime*) captures the behaviors of the subject during the various phases of the swallowing act. The fourth section (*Ii4s correction*) includes the scores of the first three sections and identifies additional information collected by the examiner and not subjected to scoring. The MAS is usually administered by a speech therapist. Another tool for analyzing behavior during meals is the *Mealtime Assessment Tool* (MAT) (Rossi et al. 2020), which is a tool for quantitative and qualitative analysis of meals (see *Appendix, Card C*). The MAT is an abbreviated and quantitative version of the *Meal Observation Grid* (Amitrano and Crinelli 2005). The scale consists of 12 items that investigate the different behaviors observable during a meal. The meal that is observed is generally lunch or dinner, which, in our culture, are the longest meals. If information on other meals is needed, this tool can be used with equal reliability. The MAT is a validated tool and was conceived by the authors as a practical guide for meal observation for nonprofessionals. In this way, it was intended to mitigate a major limitation of such observation tests, that is, the duration, which prevents widespread use by professionals. Indeed, as often mentioned, the observation lasts the entire meal and takes place in natural situations, which means that in a facility, the therapist can administer only one test a day, since patients generally consume the meal simultaneously or at very close times. The observation is carried out in a blinded manner, and in this case, the administration by the usual caregiver offers undoubted advantages for the "masking" of the examiner. The scale consists of 12 items that investigate the different aspects observable during a meal. The answers to the questions are preset alternatives, and each is assigned a score from 0 to 5, which indicates the best performance. The sum of the scores obtained for the individual items constitutes the total score. Additionally, in this test, the examiner is asked to indicate the duration of the meal: this is a data that does not contribute to the score, but it is a useful element that allows the clinician to make inferences about meal consumption. How much the patient actually consumes during a meal is an essential element for the important nutritional impact on the patient's general health and, indirectly, swallowing functionality. To detect how much of the provided dishes the patient actually eats, a specific food diary for dysphagic patients has been developed (see *Appendix, Card D*). The food diary of patients with dysphagia (Matino 2013) is not classifiable as a true evaluation tool, as none of the information collected provides knowledge about the swallowing ability of the subject. This food diary serves to monitor the actual amounts that the subject takes and is particularly useful in patients followed at home, with no direct control by health personnel, as opposed to hospitalized subjects. The diary can be filled out directly by the subject or by the caregiver or both, a condition that allows us to assess the patient's reliability. In the different columns of the diary, the compiler is asked to indicate the meal to which the observation refers, the presence or absence of cough episodes, and the portions actually consumed, by coloring the slices of the typical circle of food diaries.

References

Amitrano A, Crinelli V. The observation grid of behavior during the meal of the dysphagic patient. Logopedia e Comunicazione. 2005;1(1):49–58.

Amitrano A, Pezzella FR. The evaluation of dysphagia: development of a new scale of risk of malnutrition and pneumonia ab ingestis. Logopedia e Comunicazione. 2009;5(2):145–51.

Amitrano A, Rossi G, Acquaviva G, Fabbri S, Anticoli S, Burani N, Felzani G, Galeoto G, Ruoppolo G, Pezzella FR. Dysphagia Risk Score two (DRS2): development and validation of a rapid screening card for dysphagia in patients with stroke. Audiologia e Foniatria. 2023;8(1):34–42. https://doi.org/10.14658/pupj-IJAP-2023-1-5.

ASHA (American Speech-Language-Hearing Association). National Outcome Measurement System (NOMS): adult speech-language pathology training manual. Rockville: ASHA; 1998.

Battel I, Ceolin A, Koch I, Ventura L, Tonin P, Palmer K, Meneghello F. Comparison of the cough reflex test and water swallowing test in healthy participants and neurological patients. B-ENT. 2016;12(4):285–9.

Battel I, Calvo I, Walshe M. Cross-cultural validation of the Italian version of the functional oral intake scale. Folia Phoniatr Logop. 2018;70(3–4):117–23. https://doi.org/10.1159/000490792.

Birchall O, Bennett M, Lawson N, Cotton S, Vogel AP. Fiberoptic endoscopic evaluation of swallowing and videofluoroscopy swallowing assessment in adults in residential care facilities: a scoping review protocol. JBI Evid Synth. 2020;18(3):599–609. https://doi.org/10.11124/JBISRIR-D-19-00015.

Carnaby-Mann G, Lenius K. The bedside examination in dysphagia. Phys Med Rehabil Clin N Am. 2008;19(4):747.

Cichero JA, Heaton S, Bassett L. Triaging dysphagia: nurse screening for dysphagia in an acute hospital. J Clin Nurs. 2009;18(11):1649–59. https://doi.org/10.1111/j.1365-2702.2009.02797.x.

Clavé P, Arreola V, Romea M, Medina L, Palomera E, Serra-Prat M. Accuracy of the volume-viscosity swallow test for clinical screening of oropharyngeal dysphagia and aspiration. Clin Nutr. 2008;27(6):806–15. https://doi.org/10.1016/j.clnu.2008.06.011.

Cot F, Desharnais G. Dysphagia in adults. Paris: Maloine; 1985.

Crary MA, Mann GD, Groher ME. Initial psychometric assessment of a functional oral intake scale for dysphagia in stroke patients. Arch Phys Med Rehabil. 2005;86(8):1516–20. https://doi.org/10.1016/j.apmr.2004.11.049.

DePippo KL, Holas MA, Reding MJ. Validation of the 3-oz water swallow test for aspiration following stroke. Arch Neurol. 1992;49(12):1259–61. https://doi.org/10.1001/archneur.1992.00530360057018.

Donovan NJ, Daniels SK, Edmiaston J, Weinhardt J, Summers D, Mitchell PH, American Heart Association Council on Cardiovascular Nursing and Stroke Council. Dysphagia screening: state of the art: invitational conference proceeding from the state-of-the-art nursing symposium, international stroke conference 2012. Stroke. 2013;44(4):e24–31. https://doi.org/10.1161/STR.0b013e3182877f57.

Fattori B, Giusti P, Mancini V, Grosso M, Barillari MR, Bastiani L, Molinaro S, Nacci A. Comparison between videofluoroscopy, fiberoptic endoscopy and scintigraphy for diagno-

sis of oro-pharyngeal dysphagia. Acta Otorhinolaryngol Ital. 2016;36(5):395–402. https://doi.org/10.14639/0392-100X-829.
Firino A, Raimondo S. Cervical auscultation and pulse oximetry monitoring in the clinical evaluation of oropharyngeal dysphagia. Update of the literature. Logopedia e Comunicazione. 2019;15(3):395–414.
Foley NC, Martin RE, Salter KL, Teasell RW. A review of the relationship between dysphagia and malnutrition following stroke. J Rehabil Med. 2009;41(9):707–13. https://doi.org/10.2340/16501977-0415.
Gatti R. What is experimental pedagogy. Rome: Carocci; 2002.
Katzan IL, Cebul RD, Husak SH, Dawson NV, Baker DW. The effect of pneumonia on mortality among patients hospitalized for acute stroke. Neurology. 2003;60(4):620–5. https://doi.org/10.1212/01.wnl.0000046586.38284.60.
Kwon S, Sim J, Park J, Jung Y, Cho KH, Min K, Kim M, Kim JM, Im SH. Assessment of aspiration risk using the Mann assessment of swallowing ability in brain-injured patients with cognitive impairment. Front Neurol. 2019;10:1264. https://doi.org/10.3389/fneur.2019.01264.
Lambert HC. The McGill Ingestive skills assessment (mIsA-I). Italian version. Milan: FrancoAngeli; 2011.
Lambert HC, Gisel EG, Groher ME, Wood-Dauphinee S. McGill Ingestive Skills Assessment (MISA): development and first field test of an evaluation of functional ingestive skills of elderly persons. Dysphagia. 2003;18(2):101–13. https://doi.org/10.1007/s00455-002-0091-2.
Leder SB, Espinosa JF. Aspiration risk after acute stroke: comparison of clinical examination and fiberoptic endoscopic evaluation of swallowing. Dysphagia. 2002;17(3):214–8. https://doi.org/10.1007/s00455-002-0054-7.
Leslie P, Drinnan MJ, Finn P, Ford GA, Wilson JA. Reliability and validity of cervical auscultation: a controlled comparison using videofluoroscopy. Dysphagia. 2004;19(4):231–40.
Logemann J. Evaluation and treatment of swallowing disorders. Austin: Pro-Ed; 1983.
Logemann JA, Veis S, Colangelo L. A screening procedure for oropharyngeal dysphagia. Dysphagia. 1999;14(1):44–51. https://doi.org/10.1007/PL00009583.
Mann G. The Mann assessment of swallowing ability, vol. 1. New York: Cengage Learning; 2002.
Martino R, Foley N, Bhogal S, Diamant N, Speechley M, Teasell R. Dysphagia after stroke: incidence, diagnosis, and pulmonary complications. Stroke. 2005;36(12):2756–63. https://doi.org/10.1161/01.STR.0000190056.76543.eb.
Martino R, Silver F, Teasell R, Bayley M, Nicholson G, Streiner DL, Diamant NE. The Toronto Bedside Swallowing Screening Test (TOR-BSST): development and validation of a dysphagia screening tool for patients with stroke. Stroke. 2009;40(2):555–61. https://doi.org/10.1161/STROKEAHA.107.510370.
Matino E. Food diary: possible use in outpatient treatment of dysphagia, Unpublished thesis, University of Tor Vergata, Rome; 2013.
McCullough GH, Martino R. Clinical evaluation of patients with dysphagia. In: Shaker R, editor. Manual of diagnostic and therapeutic techniques for disorders of deglutition. New York: Springer; 2013.
Mozzanica F, Scarponi L, Pedrali S, Pizzorni N, Pinotti C, Foieni F, Zuccotti G, Schindler A. Dysphagia screening in subacute care settings using the Italian version of the Royal Brisbane and Women's Hospital (I-RBWH) dysphagia screening tool. Acta Otorhinolaryngol Ital. 2017;37(1):25–31. https://doi.org/10.14639/0392-100X-1057.
O'Neil KH, Purdy M, Falk J, Gallo L. The dysphagia outcome and severity scale. Dysphagia. 1999;14(3):139–45. https://doi.org/10.1007/PL00009595.
Oh JC, Park JH, Jung MY, Yoo EY, Chang KY, Lee TY. Relationship between quantified instrumental swallowing examination and comprehensive clinical swallowing examination. Occup Ther Int. 2016;23(1):3–10. https://doi.org/10.1002/oti.1391.
Rosenvinge SK, Starke ID. Improving care for patients with dysphagia. Age Ageing. 2005;34(6):587–93. https://doi.org/10.1093/ageing/afi187.

Rossi G, Galeoto G, Amitrano A, Berardi A, Tofani M, Celletti C, Camerota F. Development and validation of a new mealtime assessment tool (MAT) for patients with dysphagia: a cross sectional study. Clin Ter. 2020;171(4):e346–56.

Sessler CN, Gosnell MS, Grap MJ, Brophy GM, O'Neal PV, Keane KA, Tesoro EP, Elswick RK. The Richmond Agitation-Sedation Scale: validity and reliability in adult intensive care unit patients. Am J Respir Crit Care Med. 2002;166(10):1338–44. https://doi.org/10.1164/rccm.2107138.

Trapl M, Enderle P, Nowotny M, Teuschl Y, Matz K, Dachenhausen A, Brainin M. Dysphagia bedside screening for acute-stroke patients: the Gugging Swallowing Screen. Stroke. 2007;38(11):2948–52. https://doi.org/10.1161/STROKEAHA.107.483933.

Troll C, Trapl-Grundschober M, Teuschl Y, Cerrito A, Compte MG, Siegemund M. A bedside swallowing screen for the identification of post-extubation dysphagia on the intensive care unit—validation of the Gugging Swallowing Screen (GUSS)-ICU. BMC Anesthesiol. 2023;23(1):122. https://doi.org/10.1186/s12871-023-02072-6.

Valentini D, et al. MAs. Mealtime Assessment Scale. Speech therapy evaluation protocol at mealtime. Turin: Edizioni Libreria Cortina; 2015.

Treatment of Dysphagia in Adult Dysphagic Patients

4

Treatment is the natural continuation of the evaluation of swallowing in cases where difficulties are found. In terms of swallowing and oral feeding, two key concepts should be considered: safety and nutritional effectiveness. By safety, we refer to the neutralization of the risk that the bolus may enter the airways, increasing both the risk of choking, according to its size, and the risk of lung infection. Nutritional effectiveness, on the other hand, refers to the ability of the ingested bolus to meet the nutritional and hydration needs of the individual. The treatment of dysphagia is strongly bound by these two concepts, which determine the methods of execution and the limits of applicability. The goal of treatment is functional swallowing, that is, a para-physiological mode of swallowing with no aspiration, even if the transit times of the bolus in the oropharyngeal canal may be longer than normal and minimal residues may remain in the oral cavity (Schindler 1990) (Table 4.1). Historically, the treatment of dysphagia has been based on two different approaches: compensation and re-education. The compensatory approach includes all strategies that, while not modifying the physiology of the swallowing act, ensure the safety and functionality of swallowing. The rehabilitative approach, on the other hand, includes all strategies that affect the physiology of swallowing, achieving stable changes. In the first phase of its young history, speech therapy treatment was mainly based on the search for compensation, but today, there are techniques and tools, and above all theories, that have given a significant boost to the use of re-educational techniques. A preventive approach is also spreading, reserved for those individuals who must undergo treatments, for example, chemoradiotherapy, in which the onset of dysphagia is the expected consequence of the planned treatments. The choice of the type of approach is closely linked to the outcome of the evaluation, which is responsible for identifying the dysfunctional traits of swallowing. The use of one of the two approaches is almost never alternative, but most of the time, the rehabilitator uses both, with a different coefficient of use of the rehabilitative or compensatory approach on the basis of the phase of the rehabilitative path. In the early stages of

A. Amitrano, *Dysphagia and Nutrition*,
https://doi.org/10.1007/978-3-031-77449-2_4

Table 4.1 Physiological and functional swallowing

Physiological swallowing	Functional swallowing
Oropharyngeal transit time = 2 s	Oropharyngeal transit time >2 s
No aspiration	No aspiration
No residue in mouth and pharynx	Minimal residue in mouth and pharynx

taking charge of the dysphagic patient, the approach is predominantly compensatory, whereas during the course of therapy and with the progress of rehabilitative goals, the use of compensation is gradually reduced. Compensatory strategies, in fact, produce an immediate effect, thus quickly solving the patient's swallowing problems. The rehabilitative approach, on the other hand, produces results that are spread over time, but are more stable. Furthermore, the functional improvement, obtained via a compensation technique, is strictly dependent on the use of the technique itself; the rehabilitative approach, on the other hand, produces improvements that, at a certain point, are independent of the exercise itself (Schindler et al. 2011).

4.1 Compensation Strategies

Compensation strategies play an important role in managing patients with dysphagia. By compensation, we refer to all those strategies that allow overcoming or mitigating the effects of a problem without eliminating it. The use of compensation strategies is limited to the period in which they are necessary, and, above all, the benefits they produce are linked to the correct use of the strategy itself. The result produced by compensation strategies is immediate, as happens in the use of certain consistencies, or follows the often very short learning times of the strategy itself; when this consists of a motor program, think of swallowing with a rotated head. The compensation strategies that can be adopted are as follows:

- Postural compensation
- Dietary compensation

The first group includes all modifications of the position, mainly of the head, which, by modifying the path of the bolus inside the swallowing channel, make swallowing possible and safer. The second group includes all the modifications that the rehabilitator makes to the physical characteristics of the food to make its transit in the oropharyngolaryngeal channel possible and safer.

4.1.1 Postural Compensation

The position of the body and head during feeding affects the way and timing with which a bolus flows within the swallowing channel. In particular, the position of the body has a gravitational effect on the pharyngeal transport of the bolus and on reaching the pressure peaks in this phase (Castell et al. 1990; Ingervall and Lantz 1973). In the upright position, the force of gravity facilitates the flow of the bolus in the pharynx, which results in the fastest reaching of the pressure peaks. Conversely, in the supine position, the bolus flows more slowly, but the maximum lateral pressure peaks of the pharynx are activated (Barkmeier et al. 2002). In both these modes of swallowing, in the upright and supine positions, there are no differences in the activation of the protective musculature of the larynx (ibid). In the swallowing of dysphagic subjects, the upright trunk position is recommended to allow the bolus to take advantage of gravitational attraction. Furthermore, the upright position avoids the possible reflux of gastric contents into the esophagus (Portale et al. 2007). In the supine position, the abdominal contents exert pressure on the diaphragm, which, in turn, puts pressure on the stomach, thus favoring reflux of the gastric contents (Tutuian et al. 2003). This mass, rising along the esophagus, can reach the pharynx and then transit into the larynx, causing aspiration phenomena and consequent pulmonary inflammation (aspiration pneumonitis). The position that the head assumes in the space can modify the direction of the bolus and the dimensions of the pharynx, becoming wider or narrower in relation to the different positions of the head. The use of head postures can be conditioned by the patient's ability to learn and remember a certain position and by the physical reserve of the subject, who could be tired from the repeated use of a posture. The rehabilitator, therefore, will have to choose the most suitable posture according to the patient's difficulties but, above all, evaluate his ability to learn and memorize the posture itself and its compatibility with the individual physical reserve. Whenever possible, the choice of the optimal head posture must be made under instrumental control, to verify the effects that its variations produce on the subject's swallowing capacity (Table 4.2). Single positions can often be variously combined with each other on the basis of the specific individual needs of the patient.

The extended head posture (head extension) is achieved by asking the patient to extend the head once the bolus preparation phase is finished and to maintain this position during swallowing (Fig. 4.1). In this way, the bolus's movement inside the

Table 4.2 Head postures: indications and contraindications

Posture	Indications	Contraindications
Extended head	Absence of tongue thrust	Poor pharyngeal functionality Insufficient airway protection
Forward flexed head	Airway protection	Presence of pharyngeal residues Respiratory stress
Rotated head	Unilateral pharyngeal dysmotility and reduced opening of the SES	
Laterally flexed head	Unilateral pharyngeal dysmotility	
Flexed and rotated head	Presence of pharyngeal stagnations	

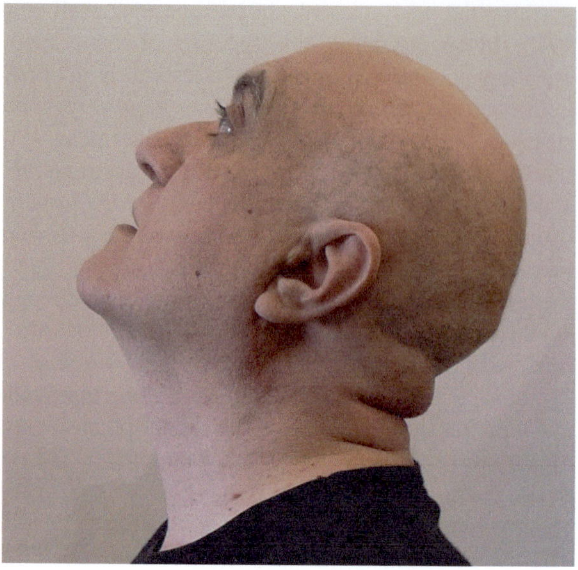

Fig. 4.1 Extended head posture

mouth is facilitated, putting it in favor of the force of gravity that attracts it to the back of the mouth. The extended head posture is used in all cases of difficulty in transporting the bolus, when the tongue cannot produce the necessary pressures to push the bolus toward the back of the mouth and the pharynx. This is the condition in which patients with hypomobility or surgical amputation of the tongue find themselves. Patients who use this posture must demonstrate adequate pharyngeal functionality and high efficiency of the airway protection system. The extended head posture also affects the opening of the upper esophageal sphincter (UES) and the coordination between breathing and swallowing (Castell et al. 1993). In fact, the extended head posture reduces the opening time of the UES, thus modifying the coordination between breathing and swallowing. An extended head posture is often contraindicated because it exposes the patient to a high risk of aspiration. The forward flexed head posture (chin tuck) is achieved by asking the patient, while swallowing, to flex his head forward almost to touch the chest with the chin (Fig. 4.2).

This posture has been proposed as a strategy to facilitate the protection of the airways during swallowing (Ekberg 1986). The anterior flexion of the head favors closure of the laryngeal vestibule (Castell et al. 1993), narrows the oropharynx (Welch et al. 1993), and reduces the distance between the hyoid bone and the larynx (Bülow et al. 2001). This forward flexion of the head does not alter the pharyngeal pressure. A weaker pharyngeal contraction was detected only in a small number of healthy subjects (Bülow et al. 1999). The duration of swallowing apnea is longer in patients whose trunk is reclined by 60° and whose head is flexed by 60°. This situation can increase respiratory stress (Ayuse et al. 2006). Several studies have reported a reduction in bolus passage in the airways, which is determined by the posture of the anterior flexed head posture (Shanahan et al. 1993; Logemann et al. 1994, 2008; Lewin et al. 2001; Terré and Mearin 2012). It has also been reported that the anterior flexed head posture does not provide benefits; and therefore, its use is discouraged in

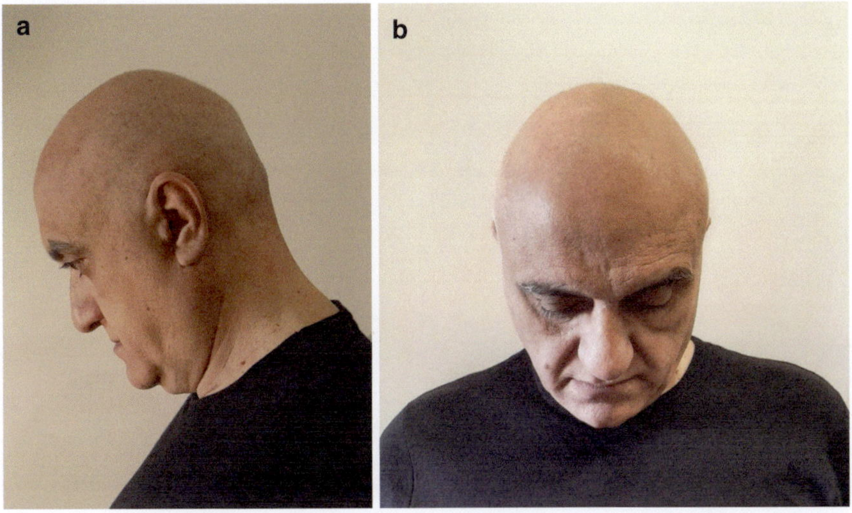

Fig. 4.2 Forward flexed head posture

subjects with delayed swallowing onset and in those with residues in the pharynx after swallowing (Shanahan et al. 1993). In summary, before the anterior flexion of the head is introduced, the rehabilitator must evaluate the general swallowing performance, the presence of residues in the pharynx, and any changes in breathing induced by this posture. The rotated head posture (head turn) is achieved by asking the patient to rotate the head to the right or left during swallowing (Fig. 4.3).

This is also a maneuver that favors swallowing, aiding the progression of the bolus in patients with unilateral pharyngeal dysmotility (Kirchner 1967; Logemann et al. 1989). The patient is asked to rotate the head from the side of the damaged hemipharynx during swallowing: in this way, the dimensions of the piriform sinus of the injured side are reduced, and the dimensions from the healthy side are widened, toward which the bolus is forced to flow. In addition, rotation of the head induces a decrease in the closure pressure of the UES, consequently prolonging the opening time of the sphincter itself (Logemann et al. 1989; McCulloch et al. 2010; Kim et al. 2015). The rotation of the head can therefore also be used in cases of reduced UES opening. The lateral flexed head posture (head tilt) is achieved by asking the patient to flex the head laterally while swallowing (Fig. 4.4). In this posture, the bolus, attracted by gravity, is forced to flow on one side only of the pharynx. In this case, the patient is asked to flex his head from the healthy side of the pharynx, excluding the hypomobile side. In other words, in the case of unilateral pharyngeal dysmotility, the rehabilitator has two compensatory options: the patient can flex the head from the healthy side or rotate the head from the hypomobile side. If the two postures are equally efficient, the patient is allowed to choose the most comfortable one. The flexed and rotated head posture (chin tuck and head turn) is achieved by asking the patient to simultaneously flex the head forward and rotate it laterally (Fig. 4.5). In this way, the distance between the cricoid cartilage and the pharyngeal wall increases, and the number of openings of the UES increases. Pharyngeal

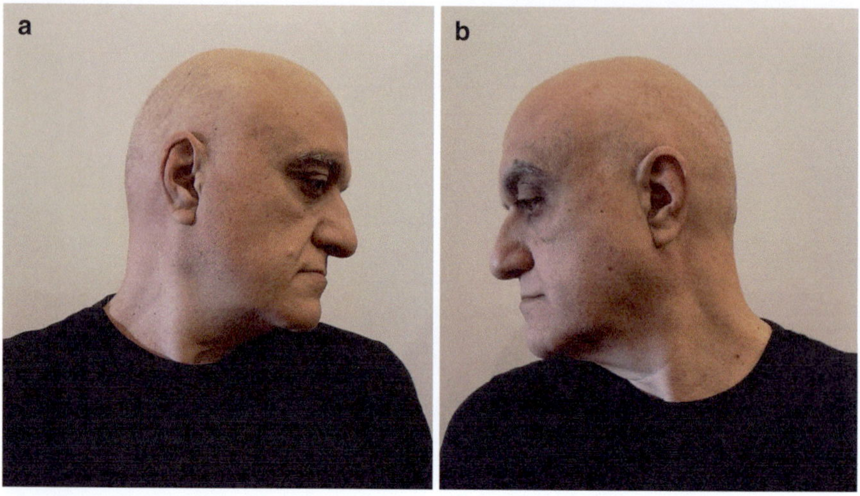

Fig. 4.3 Rotated head posture

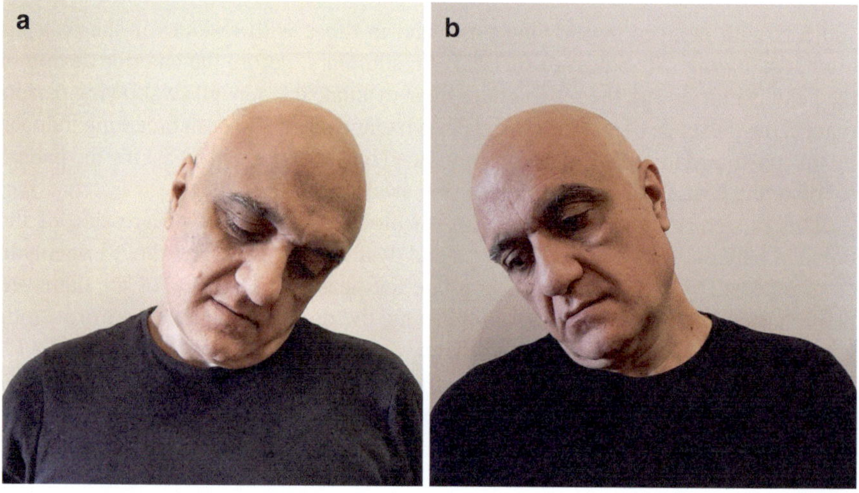

Fig. 4.4 Laterally flexed head posture

peristalsis is significantly improved. This posture has proven to be very effective in subjects with significant pharyngeal stagnation (Nagy et al. 2016).

4.1.2 Dietary Compensation

The physical characteristics of food affect the ways in which individual boluses are swallowed. The swallowing system, in fact, behaves differently, depending on whether the bolus is solid or liquid (Table 4.3). Solid foods must be efficiently

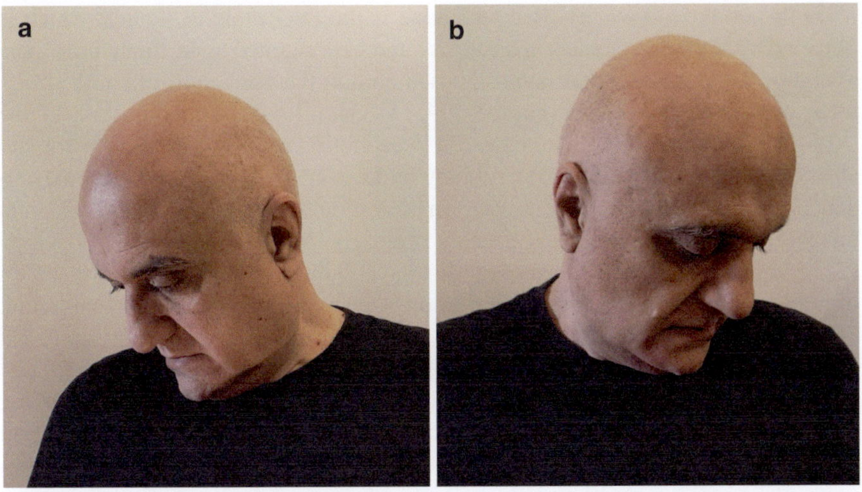

Fig. 4.5 Flexed and rotated head posture

Table 4.3 Swallowing of different consistencies

Consistency	Swallowing	Types of food
Liquids	Do not require the oral phase	Water, tea, coffee
Semiliquids	Require very little oral preparation	Drinkable yogurt
Semisolids	Require minimal oral preparation	Pudding
Solids	Require oral preparation	Pasta, bread
Soft solids	Require shorter oral preparation compared to solids	Overcooked pasta, boiled potatoes
Ground	When the individual parts are small, they require oral preparation similar to soft solids	Ground meat in tomato sauce (not meatballs)
Double consistencies	Very complex oral preparation	Small pasta in broth, ripe fruit or with juice, toasted slices in milk or tea

prepared to flow in the swallowing channel without causing damage to the channel itself. In this sense, mastication can be understood as the process that, within the mouth, gives food the necessary modifications to flow in the swallowing channel. In fact, the bolus is broken down and reduced into smaller parts, which, owing to the role of saliva, are reassembled to be then swallowed. The bolus is modified in its volumetric characteristics by the teeth and in its thermal characteristics by saliva, which regulates its temperature, making it suitable for descent along the swallowing channel. Using dietary compensation strategies, the characteristics of boluses are modified to facilitate their safe flow in the swallowing channel (Pardoe 1993). The rehabilitator therefore adjusts the consistency of the food to the specific difficulties of the patient (O'Gara 1990). For example, patients with difficulty in the oral preparation phase are fed semiliquid or semisolid foods, which, by their nature, require little oral preparation.

In this context, a widely used technique is the thickening of liquids, which is obtained by adding thickening substances (starches or gums) to the liquid itself. The alteration of the viscosity of liquids is used both in the evaluation and in the treatment of dysphagic patients (Pardoe 1993; O'Gara 1990). A modification of the swallowing mechanisms and a reduction in aspiration result from the different viscosities (Kuhlemeier et al. 2001). A study by Logemann et al. (2008) reported evidence of the effect of liquid thickening on aspiration by patients both with dementia and with Parkinson's disease. Aspiration is closely linked to the degree of thickening of liquids and to the volume of the sip. An unpublished study reported that 5 ml of liquid produces 20% aspiration if the consistency is liquid, 5% if it is semiliquid, and 5% if it is solid. With 10 ml boluses, aspiration remains at 20% for liquids but increases to 15% and 20% for semiliquids and semisolids, respectively. The residue in the valleculae, investigated with a radiological technique, also varies depending on the consistency and volume of the bolus. In particular, with a 5 ml and 10 ml liquid bolus, 65% of the residue is semiliquid, whereas with 5 ml boluses, it varies from 70% to 80% with 10 ml boluses, and with semisolids, it is 80% with boluses of 5 ml and 90% with boluses of 10 ml (Groher and Crary 2021). Notably, a reduction in the number of aspirations is not present in the last boluses (Kuhlemeier et al. 2001). This suggests a probable effect of fatigue on the patient's performance: these elements should lead the clinician to carefully evaluate the subject's swallowing ability to introduce specific elements that go beyond the simple prescription of thickening liquids. While many studies report a reduction in the number of aspirations with the use of thickened liquids (Reimers-Neils et al. 1994; Garcia et al. 2005; Kuhlemeier et al. 2001), the risk of dehydration faced by dysphagic patients who often do not accept hydration with thickened liquids (Whelan 2001) should not be overlooked. It has been estimated that approximately 50% of patients do not regularly use the thickened liquids prescribed (Shim et al. 2013). For these patients, the *Frazier Free Water Protocol* has been proposed (Panther 2008; Karagiannis and Karagiannis 2014).

This protocol was implemented in 1984 at the Frazier Rehabilitation Institute to meet the hydration needs of subjects with dysphagia who refused to take thickened liquids. Non-thickened liquids, with due caution and appropriate postural compensation, were provided before and 30 min after the end of meals, never during mealtime. In 1984, the authors noted that many patients, who, against medical advice, chose to take non-thickened liquids, did not develop pneumonia from ingestion (Panther 2008). The evidence supporting the use of the *Frazier Free Water Protocol* is still scarce, so some authors reiterate that it is inappropriate for health professionals to use methods not supported by scientific evidence (Coyle 2011). Other authors discuss the indirect evidence in support of the *Frazier Free Water Protocol* (Langmore 2011; Scibilia et al. 2016; Gillman et al. 2017). First there is poor acceptance by patients of thickened liquids, with the consequent risk of dehydration and the finding that, even in the presence of tube feeding, aspiration pneumonia can occur. Moreover, water aspirated in small quantities is relatively benign (Feinberg et al. 1990), whereas thickened liquids, if aspirated, pose a greater risk than non-thickened water (Holas et al. 1994). In the absence of strong evidence, the use of the

Frazier Free Water Protocol remains limited to selected cases, in which the clinician is called upon to make decisions on the basis of the best available evidence, their own experience, and the patient's will. Similarly, the *Ice Chip Protocol* (Pisegna and Langmore 2018) is based on the poor propensity, in the absence of concomitant causes, of aspirated water to cause pneumonia from ingestion (Feinberg et al. 1990, 1996; Langmore 2001; Olson 1970; Robbins et al. 2008; Simonelli et al. 2010; Splaingard et al. 1988). The protocol, which consists of administering crushed ice, alerts patients with good oral hygiene and is able to maintain a sitting position. The individual ice flakes are approximately 5 × 7 mm in size and correspond to a volume of melted water of approximately 1 ml. The patient is given a small spoonful of crushed ice with the instructions to chew it and then swallow it. The *Ice Chip Protocol* serves to assess the swallowing ability of patients on a nil per os regimen and to stimulate, in the same patients, swallowing, which generally slows down. In fact, patients on a nil per os regimen have a lower swallowing frequency than those who eat orally (Crary and Groher 2006). A subject who eats orally on a regular basis swallows approximately 1–4 times per minute (Langmore 2001; Murray et al. 1996). The number of swallows per unit of time decreases in subjects fed via a nasogastric tube until it disappears, or it becomes occasional in subjects on a nil per os regimen. Patients with reduced or absent swallowing are ideal candidates for the *Ice Chip Protocol*, which, although in need of further studies, has proven useful in reducing pharyngeal secretions and weaning patients from NG feeding.

Other characteristics, in addition to consistency, can be used to increase the patient's ability and safety in swallowing liquids.

Bülow et al. (2003) reported that, in patients with neurogenic dysphagia, the intake of carbonated water at volumes of 5 and 10 ml leads to a decrease in aspiration episodes compared with non-carbonated water. This is possible owing to faster transit times through the pharynx and the presence of fewer residues compared with thickened liquids (Larsson et al. 2017). The presence of carbonic acid, a diprotic acid that forms following the reaction of carbon dioxide with water, in carbonated water improves swallowing performance, because it stimulates chemosensitive afferents of the swallowing organs (Krival and Bates 2012). Studies on normal subjects have shown that sour, sweet, and salty liquids reduce the swallowing speed (Chee et al. 2005). Other studies (Miyaoka et al. 2006) have not reported substantial differences in the swallowing of foods with different tastes (sweet, salty, sour, bitter, and umami). Like liquids, other consistencies can be modified according to the specific difficulties of the dysphagic patient. The decision on the type of consistency suitable for feeding can be derived only from careful evaluation of the specific swallowing problem. The choice is not defined exclusively on the basis of safety but also on the ability of the chosen consistency to meet the patient's caloric and water needs. In this sense, the involvement of nutritionists and dieticians in the choice of diet type is important. Continuous monitoring of the patient's performance is also important to verify the adequacy of the diet to meet the changing needs of the clinical course. Importantly, centers that care for patients with dysphagia have specific diets: the National Dysphagia Diet Task Force (2002) has proposed the *National Dysphagia Diet* (NDD), which includes four different diet levels (Table 4.4).

Table 4.4 NDD diet levels

Level 1	Creamy diet	Homogeneous pudding-like consistency, very cohesive, requires bolus control, does not require chewing
Level 2	Diet with mechanically treated foods	Semisolid, cohesive, and moist foods that require chewing
Level 3	Advanced dysphagia diet	Soft solid foods that require greater chewing competence
Level 4	Regular diet	Contains all consistencies

Table 4.5 Diets for dysphagia

Phase 1 dysphagia diet	Blended and/or homogenized foods
Diet for phase 2 dysphagia	Soft first courses and pureed second courses
Diet for phase 3 dysphagia	Pureed first courses and soft second courses
Diet for phase 4 dysphagia	Regular first and second courses

In 2008, the Higher Institute of Health published Report 08/38, which describes a diet divided into four levels, with the merit of providing, on a weekly basis, very precise indications on foods, divided by level (Gaita et al. 2008) (Table 4.5). To improve and standardize the preparation in the context of community food for dysphagic subjects, in 2024, the Italian Institute of Standardization (UNI) drafted the standard UNI 11941: "Guidelines for the determination of the consistencies of food and beverages intended for dysphagic subjects."

The consistency of the foods referred to by the different types of diet, as well as the diagnostic procedures, does not have a univocal meaning. There is indeed extreme variability in the terminology used to describe the consistency of foods. The average lexical breadth used in each nation is extraordinary: 54 different terms for solid foods and 27 for fluids. This extreme variability in defining the consistency of foods generates significant problems, both in the re-educational and diagnostic phases. In fact, the non-univocal definition of the consistency of foods creates differences in treatment between the various settings of the clinical path of dysphagic patients. The problem exists at diagnostic level too: an Australian study (Cichero et al. 2000) highlighted how—in the preparation of barium-thickened fluids for evaluative purposes, through the modified barium meal (*Modified Barium Swallow*, MBS) method, or the thickened fluids used in videofluoroscopy (*FEES*)—the consistency is not determined in a univocal way (usually, in the study, barium was added by the radiology technician by eye until a radiopaque mixture was obtained); therefore, providing a comprehensive explanation of the real value of consistency and viscosity of the administered foods is impossible. With the aim of developing a new standardized terminology at the international level and defining descriptions of the "texture" of modified foods and thickened liquids used for people suffering from dysphagia of different ages, care contexts, and cultures, the International Initiative for the Standardization of the Diet in Dysphagia (IDDSI) was established. The IDDSI has therefore proposed a series of objectives to achieve worldwide uniformity in the terminology used to describe the various consistencies and on the various tests to allow easy analysis, both by the clinician and by any caregiver or the patient himself, about the correspondence between a certain recommended consistency level and the actual level to which the administered food belongs. Foods have been divided into ten levels according to consistency and viscosity (five for fluids and five for solids), from which an eight-level scale has been developed (Fig. 4.6). This is because the two intermediate levels are superimposable and therefore usable both for solids and fluids. Each of the levels of the scale, which ranges from 0 to 7, is defined by a number, a name, and a color. The choice of color-descriptors was determined by the intent to eliminate any difficulty for people affected by any type of color blindness. A further category included in the IDDSI proposal is transitional food, which is used in the weaning phases of dysphagic patients toward the goal of a common and unrestricted diet.

On the initiative's website (Iddsi.org), translations of the scale in various languages and explanatory material on its use are available. An important aspect of the IDDSI work is the identification of simple and specific tests for different cultures with which it is possible to classify a particular food using the values expressed by the scale. Measuring viscosity requires sophisticated instrumentation, which is not expected to be present in healthcare facilities or patients' homes. The tests indicated by the IDDSI, on the other hand, are simple and require the use of easily available and usable tools in all settings. For each level, a type of test is indicated, and for some levels, more than one is used to correctly classify the food under examination. For the five levels related to liquids and fluids (from level 0 to level 4), the flow test is performed using a standard 10 ml syringe, from which the plunger and needle have been removed, and a stopwatch. A 10 ml sample of the fluid to be tested is inserted into the syringe, the nozzle of which is closed with a finger (Table 4.6). The

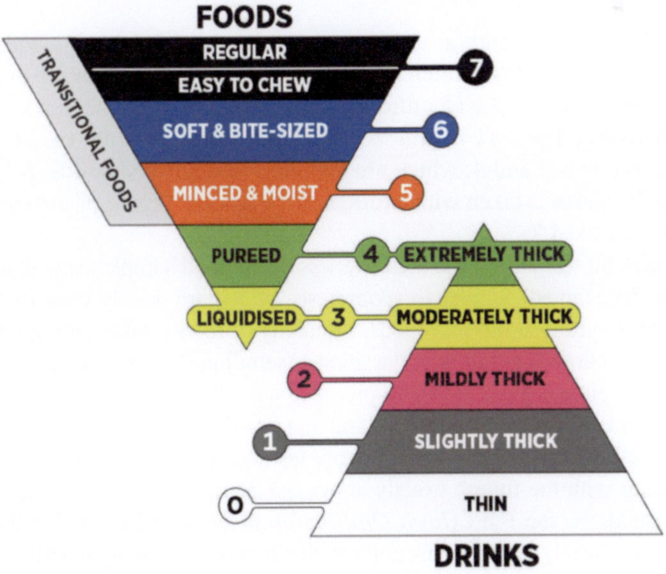

Fig. 4.6 IDDSI classification

Table 4.6 IDDSI levels identified with the flow test

Level 0 (liquid)	The liquid flows completely during the 10-second interval, leaving no residue in the graduated cylinder of the syringe
Level 1 (slightly thick)	After 10 s, a residue of 1–4 ml remains in the syringe
Level 2 (thick)	After 10 s, a residue of 4–8 ml remains in the syringe
Level 3 (moderately thick, syrupy)	More than 8 ml still contained in the syringe, but an active flow is still appreciated, even if very slow
Level 4 (very thick, creamy)	The entire content of the syringe is still present in it. The consistency could also belong to a higher level, and further tests would be necessary to verify its level with accuracy

Table 4.7 IDDSI levels identified with the *fork drip test*

Level 3 (moderately thick, syrupy)	The food drips slowly but steadily through the tines
Level 4 (very thick, creamy)	The food does not flow through the tines, but a small amount of it may drip and form drops below the utensil, which however tend not to detach

Table 4.8 IDDSI levels identified with the *spoon tilt test*

Level 3 (moderately thick, syrupy)	The sample adapts its volume to the spoon and, once tilted, drips without sticking. There may still be some residue
Levels 4 (very thick, creamy) and 5 (finely chopped, moist)	The sample maintains its shape (cohesion) and falls from the spoon without establishing any flow. It may be necessary to slightly shake the utensil to detach the food, which should leave only a minimal amount, if any, of residue

nozzle is then opened, and, at the same time, a countdown begins with the stopwatch. The nozzle is closed after 10 s: the volume still present in the syringe after this time interval allows the identification of the level of the scale in which the fluid can be classified. The *fork drip test* is used instead to describe the consistencies belonging to levels 3 and 4, which are common to fluids and solids. A quantity of the food to be tested is taken with a fork, and the amount that drips through the tines is observed (Table 4.7).

The spoon tilt test allows the adhesiveness of the food sample, as well as its cohesion, to be determined. Similar to spoon tests, which are widely used to distinguish semisolid foods from semiliquid foods, a quantity of food is taken, the spoon is tilted, and the food is allowed to fall. It is classified as semiliquid if it flows with a continuous thread and as semisolid if it falls into pieces (Table 4.8). The spoon tilt test is used to classify foods belonging to levels 3, 4, and 5: a quantity of food is taken with a spoon and then tilted on a plate. The fork pressure test consists of crushing the food with a fork, pressing with the thumb exactly above the tines, and observing the nail. It has been estimated, via the IOPI (*Iowa Oral Performance Instrument*), that the pressure needed to temporarily lose the pink color of the thumbnail, turning it white, is approximately 17 kPa, a value approximately similar to the force exerted by the tongue during swallowing. This test is used to classify foods at levels 4, 5, and 6 (Table 4.9).

Table 4.9 IDDSI levels identified with the fork pressure test

Level 4 (very thick, creamy)	Temporarily exerting force with a fork on the sample, it is possible to distinguish the marks left by the tines. Some food residues may remain between the tines
Level 5 (finely chopped, moist)	By applying pressure with a fork, the food separates easily, slipping between the tines. The food can then be crushed in this way, but the thumbnail that applies pressure should never turn white
Level 6 (tender, broken up)	The food can be easily "cut" using a fork tilted sideways. By pressing the fork on a sample of size 1.5 × 1.5 cm until the thumbnail turns white, the sample changes its shape, and there is no possibility of returning it to its original shape by removing the fork

Table 4.10 IDDSI levels identified with the spoon pressure test

Level 5 (finely chopped, moist)	The parts of the food must necessarily be smaller than 4 mm for adults and less than 2 mm for pediatric patients
Level 6 (tender, broken up)	The elements that make up the food must have a maximum size of 1.5 × 1.5 cm for adults and 8 × 8 mm for pediatric patients

The spoon pressure test has a use similar to that of the fork pressure test, which shares the administration methods and the classification levels (Table 4.10). It was introduced as a method of evaluation so as not to exclude from the use of IDDSI the populations that traditionally do not use a fork. Similarly, the *chopstick test* was developed for Asian populations that traditionally use chopsticks. The evaluation of the sample takes place, in this case, by collecting a quantity with the chopsticks, or using them to "break the sample," as happens in the fork pressure test and in the spoon pressure test. There are also populations that traditionally use their hands as the main cutlery: the *finger test* was introduced to include such populations but also to allow anyone to evaluate a sample, even in the immediate absence of suitable cutlery. The *finger test* consists of picking up a small amount of food between the thumb and index finger (Table 4.11).

The IDDSI also pays particular attention to the size of the parts that make up the foods, due to the choking risk that these constitute. Additionally, in this case, simple methods are identified to measure the individual parts. These can be measured approximately using a fork, whose average width is 1.5 cm, with a distance between two adjacent tines of approximately 2 mm. The dimensions thus defined aim to minimize the risk of choking, as each element prepared according to these indications is smaller than the glottic opening and can thus be expelled with relative ease, in the case of aspiration. Recently, level 7 (Normal) has been divided into two subclasses (7 and 7ec). The 7ec level (easy to chew) includes solid foods that can be sectioned with simple fork pressure.

This level includes everyday foods of tender consistency, without size restrictions, in relation to developmental progress and age. These foods can be consumed with any type of cutlery.

They must be free of substantial fragments, rubbery, cartilaginous, crunchy, crumbly, and fibrous (fruit and vegetables). This level can include foods and liquids of dual consistency in the presence of clinically verified safety for Level "0."

Table 4.11 IDDSI test summary

Test	IDDSI levels
Spoon pressure test	4-5-6
Fork pressure test	4-5-6
Spoon tilt test	3-4-5
Fork drip test	3-4
Flow test	0-1-2-3-4

Otherwise, the liquid consistency must be thickened according to clinical recommendations.

In addition to the eight described levels, which are related to different consistencies from liquid to solid, a broad category has been added, alongside levels 5–7, which includes the so-called transitional foods, attributable to one of the three levels they refer to and used in pediatric age to develop an awareness of chewing activity or in adulthood for the rehabilitation of the same. This category includes foods of a single consistency, which can, however, be modified through the addition of liquids (water or saliva), or with temperature variations. They require minimal or no chewing, and their structure, following changes in humidity or temperature inside the oral cavity, can be modified through tongue movements. Among dietary compensation techniques, we can also modify the feeding rhythm. Slowing down the feeding rhythm gives the subject more time to implement the motor strategies necessary for the safe swallowing of boluses. Slowing down is particularly important in impulsive patients, who tend to speed up the rhythm with which they bring food to the mouth and often increase the volume of the boluses themselves. In these cases, small spoons and cups are used for feeding, to automatically reduce the volume of the bolus.

4.2 Rehabilitative Strategies

The rehabilitative approach consists of motor stimulation to produce stable changes in the functionality of the oropharyngolaryngeal tract. In the field of deglutology, this approach has historically been less practiced than the compensatory approach. In recent years, the availability of new theoretical models and innovative instrumentation has expanded interest in the rehabilitative approach. Oromotor exercises have been widely used in speech therapy for a long period (McCauley et al. 2009). Only in recent years have studies been carried out on the effectiveness of muscle strengthening exercises in the oropharyngeal district (Robbins et al. 2005, 2007; Lazarus et al. 2003; Clark et al. 2009). Exercises for tongue strengthening have seen a significant resurgence of interest in recent years. The increase in tongue strength is correlated with better activation of the suprahyoid musculature and vertical excursion of the larynx, which results in widening of the opening of the upper esophageal sphincter (Palmer et al. 2008). Tongue strengthening exercises are among the most studied types of exercise. Motor stimulation is based on the principles of neuroplasticity, in which the exercises are programmed and executed.

4.2.1 Principles of Exercise: Neuroplasticity

The term "neuroplasticity" refers to the ability of the brain and nervous system to structurally and functionally modify themselves. This change can be induced by a series of internal and external factors (Shaw and McEachern 2001). Pascual-Leone et al. (2005) define plasticity as an intrinsic property of the central nervous system (CNS), which is active throughout the course of life and allows the brain to flexibly adapt its functional and structural organization to respond to environmental pressures, physiological changes, and experiences. There are three types of neuroplasticity:

1. *Experience expectant*, which guides brain development
2. *Experience independent*, which does not depend on experience
3. *Experience dependent*, which depends on experience

The neuroplasticity *experience expectant* manifests itself in critical periods of development and is active in defined temporal phases in which plasticity, in certain brain areas, is at its maximum in response to specific stimuli. The absence of specific environmental stimuli in critical periods of development has a negative and irreversible effect on the development of the CNS. The critical periods begin at different times of human development and have varying durations, concluding once the system has achieved stable modifications. An example is the development of ocular dominance columns of the primary visual cortex (Kandel et al. 2014).

The neuroplasticity *experience independent* is the development of the CNS independent of the external environment, which is realized following stimuli self-produced by the brain itself. An example of *independent* neuroplasticity is the development of eye-specific layers of the lateral geniculate nucleus of the cat (Campbell and Shatz 1992).

The neuroplasticity *experience dependent* is neuroplasticity dependent on modifications of the CNS in response to internal or external changes. Such plasticity is usually activated by learning processes, environmental stimuli, psychoactive drugs, and neurological and psychiatric diseases. The neuroplasticity *experience dependent* is the goal of neurorehabilitation and neuromodulation (Kolb and Gibb 2014). Initially, this type of plasticity creates rapid and reversible changes in cortical representation maps and connections between brain areas. Such modifications occur following exposures, even for short periods, to particular sensory, motor, and cognitive conditions. These transient modifications, if adequately supported and reinforced, result in the creation of new circuits that determine stable behavioral changes (Pascual-Leone et al. 2005). Motor learning is an important example of a neuroplasticity *experience dependent* process. The plasticity induced by learning is not use dependent but learning dependent. In other words, for example, it is not the generic use of a hand that induces plasticity but the use of the hand in the execution of a specific task: nonpurposeful exercise, even if intense, does not induce plasticity, and cerebral reorganization is determined by the learning of a new skill. Motor learning is specific and does not generalize to untrained motor behaviors (Krakauer 2006).

Neuroplasticity, which is *experience dependent*, does not always have a positive meaning. Sometimes, cerebral reorganization can result in unwanted consequences that become the cause of pathology, and in these cases, we speak of "maladaptive plasticity": "This maladaptive disaster reveals the dark side of cortical reorganization" (Elbert and Heim 2001, p. 139). In the field of neurorehabilitation, the goal of treatment is to promote and guide the functional recovery of the CNS after damage occurs as a result of an injurious event. The principle that guides the rehabilitator is to promote adaptive plasticity and counteract maladaptive plasticity. This is made possible with precise knowledge of the ways in which the two different processes act. In recent years, basic neuroscience has outlined the principles of *experience dependent* neuroplasticity, the application of which is indispensable in the development of neurorehabilitative treatments. The principles of neuroplasticity were defined by Kleim and Jones (2008), who described the 10 essential points to induce modifications of the CNS through experience:

1. *Use it or lose it*: not stimulating brain function leads to its functional regression.
2. *Use it and improve it*: exercise that stimulates brain function enhances it.
3. *Specificity*: the type of exercise determines the type of plasticity that will be induced. Learning does not generalize to untrained functions.
4. *Repetition*: the induction of plasticity requires repetitive exercise. The repetition of the exercise stabilizes the learned skill.
5. *Intensity*: the induction of plasticity requires intensive exercise.
6. *Time*: different forms of plasticity are activated at different stages of exercise.
7. *Salience*: exercise must be salient to induce plasticity. Attention facilitates learning.
8. *Age*: neuroplasticity is a constant characteristic throughout life. It emerges more easily in the young brain, whereas it is reduced in aging.
9. *Transference*: plasticity in response to exercise facilitates the acquisition of behavior.
10. *Interference*: plasticity in response to experience can interfere with the acquisition of another behavior.

Every rehabilitation program, in its formulation, must take into account these principles in the choice of the exercises and in the definition of training protocols. In the field of deglutology, the principles most studied thus far are those of repetitiveness, intensity, and specificity. Several studies have demonstrated the importance of the repetitiveness of exercise in producing changes (Nudo et al. 1996; Kilgard and Merzenich 1998). This repetitiveness of exercise in the field of deglutology is determined according to the criteria of progression and the acquisition of sports medicine (Robbins et al. 2005, 2007; American College of SportsMedicine 1998). With the current state of knowledge, it is not yet possible to define the optimal number of repetitions to achieve changes in the swallowing apparatus. The second most studied principle is that of intensity, i.e., the number of training sessions and their distribution over time: it has indeed been shown that intensity is important for change and the consequent result of rehabilitative treatment (Martin 2009; Carey et al. 2002).

Treatments that are too intense can have cytotoxic effects. Excitotoxicity is the process through which nerve cells can suffer damage due to excessive stimulation by neurotransmitters (Temple et al. 2001). Identifying the right intensity of exercise is therefore crucial, both for improvement and to avoid possible toxic effects. Finally, specificity characterizes the exercise that directs recovery toward a given area and pertains to the characteristic of the exercise that aims to achieve change exclusively in the neurological substrate involved in a behavior; conversely, it implies only minimal transferability to other behaviors (Kleim and Jones 2008).

4.2.2 *Isometric Progressive Resistance Oropharyngeal* (I-PRO) *Therapy*: Isometric Tongue Exercises

Isometric tongue exercises consist of tongue contractions performed without muscle stretching (Duchateau and Hainaut 1984). The contraction is obtained by opposing the tongue to a rigid and unyielding surface, which can be the hard palate, a tongue depressor, or the sensor of a pressure detector (Box 4.1).

Box 4.1 Isometric Exercise

Isometric exercise is a type of exercise that promotes muscle contraction without movement. Isometric or static contraction occurs without variation in the length of the muscle. It is obtained when the shortening of the muscle is prevented by a load equal to the muscle tension. In other words, a static contraction is obtained when the force generated by the muscle is not sufficient to move the load. In such situations, the muscle contracts but does not undergo length variations, as the load to be moved does not change. Isometric contractions are muscle contractions that are obtained by exerting pressure against an immovable and unyielding object.

Some authors have shown that isometric tongue exercises lead to improvements in the muscular strength of the tongue. Lazarus (Lazarus et al. 2003) studied a sample of young healthy subjects engaged in a program of isometric tongue exercises. The sample consisted of 30 subjects divided into 3 groups: one that did not perform the exercise program, one that performed isometric tongue exercises via the IOPI, and one that performed isometric exercises via the tongue depressor. The two groups performed the isometric exercises for four consecutive weeks, after which there was an increase in tongue strength in the two groups that had performed the isometric exercise and no increase in the group that had not performed the training protocol. Furthermore, the increase in tongue strength was substantially equal in the two groups that had practiced workouts with one technological device (IOPI) and the other with a low-technology device (tongue depressor). Robbins et al. (2005) studied a sample of ten elderly subjects, both male and female, without specific pathologies, who were engaged for eight consecutive weeks in a training program with isometric tongue exercises practiced with the aid of the IOPI. The authors noted a steady increase in tongue performance in the first 6 weeks of training, accompanied by a 5.1% increase in tongue volume, as if due to muscle hypertrophy. However, knowledge about detraining for tongue strengthening exercises is still limited (Box 4.2).

> **Box 4.2 Detraining**
> Detraining is a phenomenon that indicates the total or partial loss of physiological, anatomical, and performance adaptations related to physical exercise as a result of a variable period of reduction or absence of physical activity.

Clark et al. (2009) reported that, after 4 weeks of inactivity, healthy subjects lose the positive effects obtained in 9 weeks of training with isometric tongue exercises. In other words, the strength gained is lost in half the time it takes to acquire it. Currently, knowledge about detraining in the field of oral training is still scarce, despite its importance for the preparation of training and maintenance protocols. In the execution of isometric tongue exercises, various devices can be used to facilitate training (Figs. 4.7 and 4.8). The different devices can be divided, depending on their technological content, into the following:

- *Low-tech devices*:
  - Tongue depressors
  - Pecopanda
- *High-tech devices*:
  - IOPI (Iowa Oral Performance Instrument)
  - MOST (Madison Oral Strengthening Therapeutic)

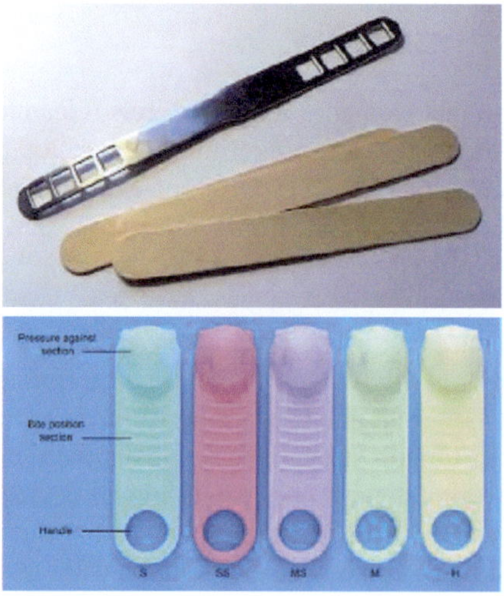

Fig. 4.7 Low-tech device

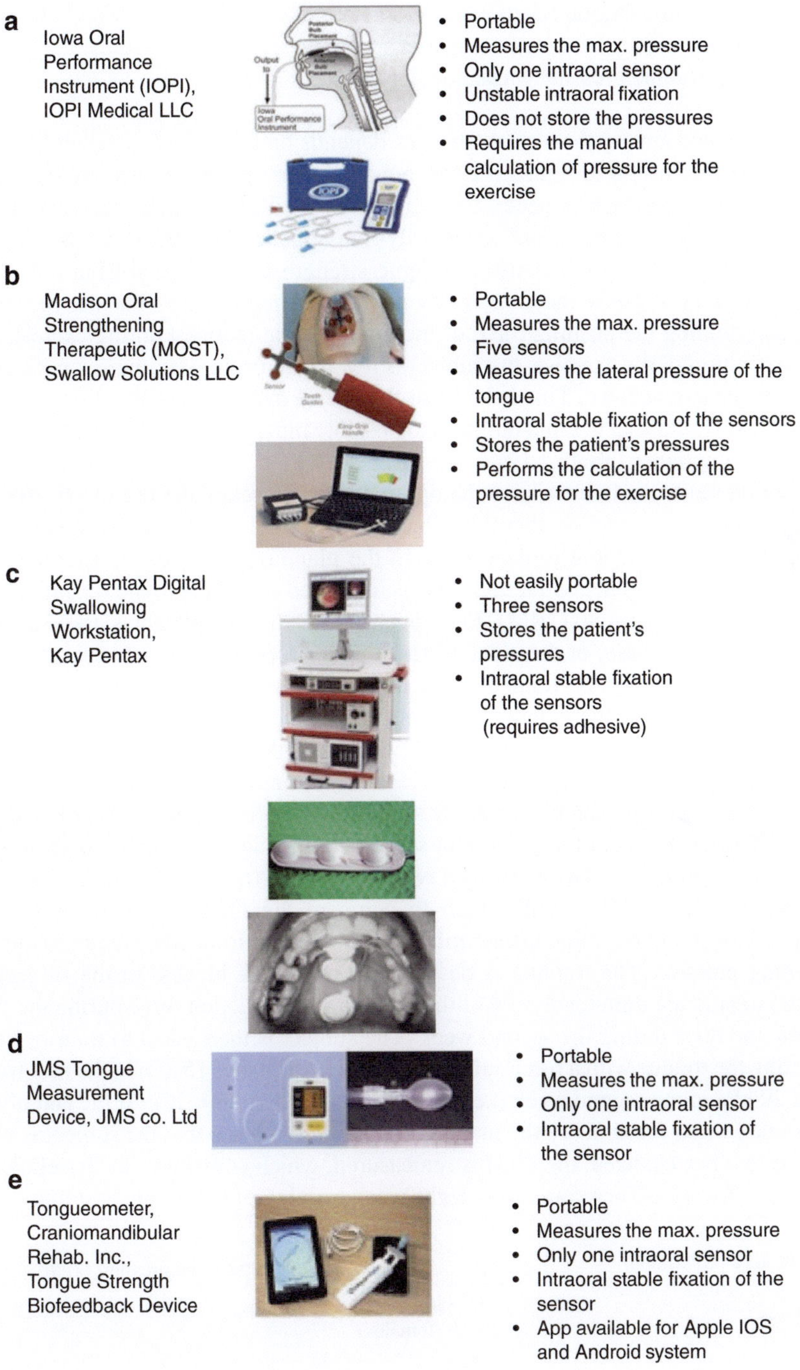

Fig. 4.8 High-tech device

- Kay Pentax Digital Swallowing Workstation
- Tongueometer
- JMS Tongue Pressure Measurement Device

The choice among the various devices depends on ease of use, availability, and cost. It is also useful to remember that not all the devices mentioned are usable in Europe due to the lack of necessary certifications. I-PRO therapy programs, while following a fixed scheme, are necessarily individualized for the determination of training pressures. The increase in tongue strength is established from an initial value, which is the baseline for quantifying the final improvement but also the value for determining the pushing force of the tongue to be required during exercise. In the execution of the exercise, the subject is not asked for the maximum tongue contraction he can achieve. This is because the use of maximum contraction for each repetition would lead to rapid fatigue and possibly muscle pain, factors that decrease patient compliance (Table 4.12).

Sports medicine indicates, as the optimal training value, the use of 60–80% of the maximum contraction that the subject can exert (Powers and Howley 2008). Therefore, it is essential to determine, in the planning phase of the exercise, the value of the maximum contraction. This is identified according to the scheme of the one repetition maximum (1RM) (Fiatarone et al. 1990). The patient is asked to contract the tip, the base, or the sides of the tongue, depending on which part of the tongue is intended to be trained, three times consecutively. If the maximum and minimum values of the contraction measured in the three repetitions differ by a value less than 5%, the highest score is considered the baseline for exercise planning. In the case where this difference exceeds 5%, a new set of three measurements is performed. If, for example, the three measurements give values of 25, 24, and 24, the difference between the maximum score obtained and the minimum score is 1 (25 max-24 min = 1). The difference was 4% (1/25 = 0.04 = 4%). In this case, 25 constitutes the baseline with which to compare the final values to verify any improvement and the value to determine the contraction force to be required during training practice. The training is designed in two-week blocks, so the subject is asked to practice training at 60% of the maximum contraction force during the first week and 80% during the second week. The subject is then asked to train by contracting the tongue with a force sufficient to reach a value of 15 kPa in the first week and 20 kPa in the second week (i.e., 25 × 0.6 = 15; 25 × 0.8 = 20). At the end of the 2 weeks, when presumably the maximum contraction force that the subject is able to express has changed, the 1RM is remeasured, which constitutes the baseline for the next 2 weeks. Therefore, in an eight-week training program, the baseline value

Table 4.12 Maximum tongue pressures in healthy subjects

Age	Maximum tongue pressure (kPa)	
20–59 (males)	45	± 10
20–59 (females)	37	± 9
Over 60	38	± 9
Over 70	32	± 9

Source: Dysphagia Team of Seirei, Fujishima (2011)

is determined at the third, fifth, and seventh weeks. The training program includes the number of repetitions within each session, as well as the number of daily training sessions and their total duration.

The various studies on oropharyngeal exercises are not uniform in indicating the number of exercise repetitions for each training session, so we have various indications of the number of isometric contractions to be performed, which vary from 10 to 30 in different protocols. Each single contraction is maintained for a time that varies from 1 to 3 s. Similarly, there are no unambiguous indications of the number of weekly training days, which can vary from one to seven (Robbins et al. 2005, 2007; Lazarus et al. 2003; Clark et al. 2009). Additionally, the duration of the training period varies from one author to another. Improvements are reported in trainings lasting 4 weeks (Lazarus et al. 2003). Other authors report improvements in longer periods, i.e., 8 or 9 weeks (Robbins et al. 2005, 2007; Clark et al. 2009), "the Robbins" protocol involves 10 tongue contractions of a single duration of 3 s, which are repeated three times a day for 3 days a week for a period of 8 weeks. Importantly, during the execution of the exercises, the feedback provided by the speech therapist to the patient should promote self-feedback, thus making the patient gradually more capable of self-monitoring (Box 4.3).

Box 4.3 The Feedback

In technical-scientific language, feedback refers to the process by which the result from the action of a system is reflected in the system itself to correct or modify its behavior. In linguistic and psychological terms, feedback is the retroactive effect of a message or an action on the one who produced it.

In the rehabilitative and sports fields, there are two types of feedback:

1. Feedback on performance
2. Feedback on the result

Feedback on performance is given by the therapist on the ways in which the subject performs the exercise.

Feedback on the result can be given by the therapist or directly detected by the patient on the device's display.

The use of devices, especially high-tech devices, is therefore important in this particular sector of swallowing rehabilitation. The devices do not seem to significantly alter the outcome of the treatment (Lazarus et al. 2003), but they influence patient compliance, which is often not easy to achieve in the execution of repetitive and not very stimulating exercises. Ultimately, the use of a device with greater technological content favors two important aspects of therapy:

1. Exercise planning
2. Feedback

4.2.3 Rehabilitation Protocols

Specific protocols have been prepared on the basis of the assumptions of neuroplasticity and motor learning. Among these, intensive dysphagia rehabilitation (IDR) (Malandraki et al. 2016) is an intensive individualized treatment based on the combination of the principles of exercise physiology, neuroplasticity, and motor learning. Preliminary results of a study on the application of the method related to a group of 10 patients have been published, in which an improvement in the scores obtained at the PAS (penetration aspiration scale) was found. Among the five patients initially fed by tube, two recovered from oral feeding, and two recovered oral feeding; only one patient experienced no significant progress in oral feeding. The initial conclusions indicate that the IDR approach is safe and improves the swallowing ability of dysphagic subjects. Further studies, which are currently being conducted at the *Purdue I-EaT Research Lab*, are necessary for the large-scale application of the method.

Another protocol is the *McNeill Dysphagia Therapy Program* (MDTP) (Carnaby-Mann and Crary 2008, 2010), named after Hannibal McNeill, who, in 2004, was the first volunteer patient for a research program on dysphagia therapy. McNeill suffers from dysphagia following a procedure at the base of the tongue and a subsequent stroke. At the beginning of the treatment, he followed a mixed diet which, after the experimental treatment, was replaced by a regular diet that he was able to maintain until his death, which occurred following a second cerebral hemorrhage. The MDTP is a systemic rehabilitation program for dysphagia that uses swallowing as an exercise. The information taken during the evaluation describes the patient's basic abilities, from which a program of specific training is built, in which swallows constitute the unit of exercise. The modification of the swallows obtained on the basis of variations in consistency and volume constitutes the criterion for load variation, which is progressively intensified. Each training session, carried out both in the clinic and at the patient's home, aims at the swallowing of a 100 boluses. The method involves 15 training sessions lasting an hour, spread over 5 days, for a period of 3 weeks. The training sessions are carried out with the simultaneous use of indirect electrical stimulation. The MDTP requires a good cognitive level in patients and is not applicable in patients with very severe dysphagia. This reaffirms the concept, as it occurs in common clinical experience, that not all dysphagia is rehabilitable.

Improvements in swallowing have been reported in patients with Parkinson's disease following the application of *Lee Silverman Voice Treatment* (LSVT). This is a method used to improve the voice in patients with Parkinson's disease on the basis of intensive voice training. One study reported improvements in swallowing functionality in a group of patients with Parkinson's disease who had undergone 4 weeks of training with LSVT (El Sharkawi et al. 2002). The videofluoroscopic study, carried out before and after the month of treatment with LSVT, revealed the following:

- The reduction in the percentage of oral residue
- The reduction in oral transit time (oral transit time, OTT)
- Increase the efficiency of the oropharyngeal phase (oropharyngeal swallow efficiency, OPSE)

The Consensus Conference in Milan (Schindler et al. 2021) on the treatment of Parkinson's disease does not include the LSVT® method among the primary treatments for dysphagia in patients with Parkinson's disease; this method is exclusively used for the treatment of voice disorders.

Increases in swallowing functionality are also reported in patients who have undergone training with expiratory muscle strength training (EMST) (Hutcheson et al. 2018; Troche et al. 2010). The expiratory muscle strengthening training is carried out by asking the patient to exhale into a one-way device, which has a resistance valve whose opening threshold can be adjusted in percentage of the individual's maximum expiratory pressure (MEP). Once the MEP is measured, exercises are performed at different percentages of the initial MEP. For example, six repetitions are performed with the valve at 70% of the MEP to be repeated for eight series, twice a day, three times a week for eight consecutive weeks. At the end of the second, fourth, and sixth weeks, the MEP is reassessed to define the new baseline from which to define the training load. The authors related the improvement in swallowing performance to the following:

- Improvement in afferent stimuli from the peripheral receptors of the tongue and palate
- Increased elevation of the hyolaryngeal complex due to greater contraction of the suprahyoid and laryngeal elevator muscles
- Greater contraction of the lateral cricoarytenoid muscles, with consequently greater efficiency of the glottic valve and the palatal elevator muscles, and improvement of the velopharyngeal valve
- Improving expiratory pressure during coughing

4.2.4 Functional Stimulation (Skill-Based Rehabilitation)

Functional stimulation is a type of motor stimulation in which individual movements are not considered but motor acts or actions, preferably in an ecological condition. In other words, with functional stimulation, the patient is not asked to open and close the mouth but, for example, to welcome different sizes and shapes with the lips. In this way, the stimulation is more motivating and ecological and above all manages to stimulate the muscular components actually involved in performing a certain motor behavior. The work is carried out on motor acts and not on individual movements (Box 4.4).

Box 4.4 The Movement

Movement: This is the result of the activation of a limited muscular district that produces displacement in the space of one or more joints.

Motor act: This is the result of several movements performed synergistically and fluidly, involving multiple joints. Unlike movements, motor acts are characterized by a purpose.

Action: Action is a sequence of motor acts characterized by a general purpose.

Therefore, we do not talk about re-education of the tongue, lips, etc., but about re-education of the different phases that, as a whole, constitute the act of swallowing. Functional stimulation, in some way, is the formalization of a statement by Jeri Logemann, according to which "the best treatment for swallowing is swallowing" (Logemann 1999). Motor exercise is no longer an active and passive stimulation of specific organs according to their own directions of movement but rather a real situation in which the different organs are engaged in simplified and protected swallowing activities as necessary. Some authors have extended this statement to declare that "oral motor exercises are not recommended for the rehabilitation of swallowing" (Cichero and Murdoch 2006). The so-called oral praxis maintains its validity in the prevention of scar retractions in patients undergoing surgical procedures in the head-neck district (Clark 2003). A functional approach to swallowing rehabilitation cannot disregard the identification, by the speech therapist, of the area of swallowing to improve. Therefore, rehabilitation must be preceded by evaluation to identify aspects of the act of swallowing that need functional improvement:

- Rehabilitation during the oral phase
- Rehabilitation of the pharyngeal phase
- Rehabilitation during both phases of swallowing
- Rehabilitation of the breathing-swallowing coordination

Each of the previous phases is a macroarea, further divisible into individual functional components.

- Oral phase:
  - Open the mouth to accept the bolus.
  - Take the bolus from a cup, spoon, or fork.
  - Close the lips to contain the bolus.
  - Manipulate a solid bolus in the oral cavity.
  - Control a liquid bolus.
  - Control a mixed bolus.
  - Move a bolus toward the pharynx.
  - Modify pressures in the mouth.
  - Collect residues.

- Pharyngeal phase:
  - Closure of the palatine veil.
  - Laryngeal excursion.
  - Transport of the bolus toward the esophagus.
  - Opening of the upper esophageal sphincter.
  - Closure of the larynx.

On the basis of the evaluation, the speech therapist can decide to work on aspects of the oral phase, on those of the pharyngeal phase, on both, or still on the coordination of breathing-swallowing or on the removal of food residues from the mouth or pharynx. From this perspective, individual exercises are incorporated within a functional problem that the swallowing apparatus must solve from time to time.

4.2.5 Biofeedback

Biofeedback, or biological feedback, is a therapeutic technique that allows individuals to learn to control and self-regulate their own physiological responses. Through biofeedback, a certain body function is monitored with the use of electrodes or transducers applied to the patient's skin. The signal captured by the electrodes is translated into an acoustic or visual signal, through which the patient can learn to control the monitored function. This extrinsic information can be considered additional information that adds to intrinsic feedback and facilitates learning, retention, and generalization of motor skills (Giggins et al. 2013; Humbert and German 2013). Biofeedback can be considered an additional method in all situations where during treatment, the patient needs to learn new motor patterns (Mulder and Hulstyn 1984). In these cases, the availability of feedback can help the subject better understand the task that is required to perform (Crary and Groher 2000). A recent systematic review reported the usefulness of using biofeedback in the treatment of swallowing disorders (Benfield et al. 2019) and in reference to the treatment of vertical motility disorders of the hyolaryngeal complex (Albuquerque et al. 2019; Benfield et al. 2019). In forced swallowing, where it is necessary to swallow using a greater force than normal, the positioning of surface electrodes can help the patient understand and perform better swallowing acts in the required mode. Importantly, biofeedback, as an exclusive technique, has no therapeutic meaning but is considered an additional technique, which can help in the execution of a therapeutic protocol. Patients with dysphagia and Parkinson's disease have proven to be particularly sensitive to treatment with biofeedback (Maas et al. 2008; Battel et al. 2021).

4.2.6 Indirect Electrical Stimulation

In recent years, electrical stimulation has been proposed to facilitate the contraction of peripheral muscles. The application of an electric current, in fact, facilitates contraction of the muscles when the peripheral nerves that innervate them are intact. Electrical stimulation has been proposed according to two different techniques: neuromuscular electrical stimulation (NMES) and pharyngeal electrical stimulation (PES).

4.2.6.1 Neuromuscular Electrical Stimulation (NMES)

An NMES system produces an electrical stimulus that, through the skin, reaches the motor end plates and, if correctly applied, activates the muscles or muscle groups in patients who do not contract them voluntarily, causing depolarization of the nerve and subsequent activation of the innervated muscle fibers.

The therapeutic benefit of electrical stimulation is linked to the contraction of skeletal muscle, with effects on strength, reaction time, and endurance.

Neuromuscular electrical stimulation is performed through surface electrodes, if transcutaneous, or inserted into the muscle, if percutaneous: in the first case, the electrodes are positioned on the submental region, and the different ways of positioning them in this area are determined by the choice of muscles to be stimulated. A generic position on the neck is absolutely to be avoided owing to the risk of stimulating the carotid sinus or causing a laryngeal spasm.

The basic parameters for the application of electrical stimulation are as follows:

- Chronaxie
- Frequency
- Intensity
- Impedance

Chronaxie is the minimum stimulation time for the target organ to be excited. Unlike for various tissues, for the oropharyngeal district, the chronology is included within an interval ranging from 100 to 300 ms. The frequency, i.e., the number of pulses per second used to stimulate the motor neurons, must instead be between 50 and 80 Hz. The intensity of the current expresses the amount of electric charge that passes through the section of a conductor in the unit of time and is measured in amperes. The variation in the intensity of the current changes the number of motor units involved: as the intensity increases, the penetration arc of the electric beam in the corresponding tissues to the position of the electrode increases. The amperage provided must promote a useful but comfortable contraction: too little amperage does not determine the degree of contraction, whereas excessive amperage can cause painful contractions or cramps. In determining the stimulation protocol, the optimal current must be defined, that is, the level of intensity suitable for stimulating the contraction of the target muscles without causing pain. Impedance is the resistance that each tissue opposes to the passage of current and depends on the type of skin and its thickness, the subcutaneous nature, and the presence of adipose tissue. Temporary factors also influence impedance, such as skin moisture, which varies with sweating, and the degree of blood perfusion. NMES cannot be applied in all patients, as it is contraindicated in individuals with pacemakers, superficial or plantar metal implants, a history of heart disorders or convulsive disorders, skin lesions, or tumors or during pregnancy. The presence of scars or tracheotomy is also a further contraindication.

In 1985, the US Food and Drug Administration (FDA) required several warning labels on neuromuscular electrical stimulation devices for severe muscle spasms of the larynx and pharynx that can occur when the electrodes are placed over the neck or mouth. These contractions can be intense enough to close the airways and cause breathing difficulties.

On June 6, 2001, the FDA granted approval for the use of a specific device, VitalStim, for the rehabilitation of dysphagia. The recognition also came with the obligation of some warnings: "The long-term effects of chronic electrical stimulation are unknown. Stimulation should not be applied over the carotid sinus nerves. If the electrodes are placed improperly and the unit is not used with the recommended frequency and intensity, it can cause laryngeal or pharyngeal spasm."

The use of NMES in the field of deglutology is still debated. However, numerous studies have reported positive results following its use in the rehabilitation of dysphagia patients (Carnaby-Mann and Crary 2008; Freed et al. 2001; Leelamanit et al. 2002; Blumenfeld et al. 2006; Shaw et al. 2007; Oh et al. 2007; Baijens et al. 2008; Ryu et al. 2009; Kushner et al. 2013; Bhatt et al. 2015). Other studies report the absence of significant changes following the use of NMES (Kiger et al. 2006; Bülow et al. 2008; Baijens et al. 2013). The discrepancy in the studies may have been determined by the diversity of the patients, as well as the stimulation protocols used, or by the different behavioral therapy protocols employed. A meta-analysis (Tan et al. 2013) revealed that NMES does not result in significant changes compared with behavioral therapy in patients with poststroke dysphagia, whereas it results in improvements in patients with dysphagia not resulting from a stroke. In a randomized, double-blind study, Carnaby-Mann et al. (2012) compared the performance of three groups of patients with poststroke dysphagia followed in the postacute phase. One group was treated with MDTP and NMES, and the other group was treated with MDTP and sham NMES, a third traditional therapy. The patients who underwent MDTP and sham NMES treatment reported the best results. On the basis of this evidence, the authors deduced the non-significance of NMES in the recovery of poststroke dysphagia patients. To the best of our knowledge, NMES is considered a promising method, but further studies are needed for the treatment of dysphagia (Groher and Crary 2021).

4.2.6.2 Pharyngeal Electrical Stimulation (PES)

PES is a new technique that stimulates pharyngeal sensory afferents. Through a probe that is introduced through the nasal cavity, electrodes are positioned near the pharynx. The intensity of the stimulation depends on the patient's sensitivity and the maximum tolerated thresholds (Restivo and Hamdy 2018). After approximately 20 years of research on PES by Professor Hamdy's group, which demonstrated the effectiveness and safety of this type of stimulation in the treatment of dysphagia, a specific commercial device for PES has been developed and is now available. The device is called Phagenyx, produced by Phagenesis Ltd. in Manchester, UK, and consists of a base station and a treatment catheter, which, if used in combination, allows the specialist to perform customized treatments for dysphagic patients.

The base station provides optimal stimulation for patients and, at the same time, has a setting limited to a specific range of intensities and frequencies that have proven to be the most effective and safe in the treatment of dysphagia. The base station also records and stores patient information to avoid treatment errors. The device is portable and battery-powered and can be operated by the operator via a touch screen interface. The stimulation is delivered to the patient's pharynx through the Phagenyx catheter introduced through the nose and connected to the base station. On the outer surface of the catheter, two electrodes deliver the stimulation. Guide signs ensure that the electrodes are positioned correctly. The electrodes are usually positioned 3 cm above the upper esophageal sphincter. The catheter is also designed to incorporate an optional feeding tube that is useful for the administration of nutrition, medications, and fluids. Studies on the use of PES in clinical practice are promising, but further research is needed to assess its value in the treatment of dysphagia (Jayasekeran et al. 2010; Scutt et al. 2015; Bath et al. 2016; Dziewas et al. 2018; Suntrup et al. 2015; Takeishi et al. 2018; Vasant et al. 2016).

4.3 Maneuvers

In the management of patients with dysphagia, an important role is played by maneuvers. Over the years, the list of maneuvers available to the rehabilitator has progressively lengthened. Before proceeding with the detailed analysis of the individual maneuvers, a distinction must be made. In Table 4.13, all the maneuvers are listed consecutively because they share the same definition and are in compliance with the classification followed by various texts on dysphagia. A maneuver consists of the series of operations necessary for the operation of a device or machine, in our case, the series of operations necessary to safely perform a swallowing act. In this sense, only some are true maneuvers; for others, the definition of "exercise" would be more appropriate. In fact, only some, such as the supraglottic swallowing maneuver, are strategies that the patient must use during the meal; others, such as the Masako maneuver, are exercises and are therefore not used during the meal but exclusively as a training mode (Table 4.13).

Table 4.13 List of maneuvers divided into exercises and strategies for swallowing

Swallowing strategies (maneuvers)	Exercises
Forced swallowing	Shaker maneuver
Decomposition of the swallowing	Masako maneuver
Supraglottic swallowing	Mendelsohn maneuver
Super-supraglottic swallowing	Rapid mandibular opening maneuver
Multiple swallows	

4.3.1 The Forced Swallowing Maneuver

The forced swallowing maneuver has been proposed as a method to voluntarily increase the force needed to swallow a specific bolus. In one of the first indications for the use of the maneuver, the patient was asked to swallow as if they were swallowing a telephone directory. This object, perhaps now little known to the younger generation, when mobile telephony did not yet exist, was a large book in which all the telephone numbers of the subscribers to a city or province's landline network were listed: in large cities, the telephone directory was a large and heavy tome. Swallowing thinking of a telephone directory somehow induced the subject to use considerable force. Bülow et al. (1999) reported the reduction of the space between the hyoid bone and the mandible before the execution of a forced swallow: this reduction involves the need for a movement of raising the larynx to a lesser extent during the execution of the forced swallow. The authors did not notice an increase in pharyngeal pressures during the execution of the forced swallow. In contrast, Huckabee (Huckabee et al. 2005; Daniels and Huckabee 2008) reported an increase in the intralaryngeal pressure and a reduction in the pressure of the UES. In a further study, Hiss and Huckabee (2005) compared the activation times of the pharyngeal contraction and the opening of the UES during the execution of the forced swallow maneuver and during normal swallowing. The activation times differed between the two types of swallowing, with longer activation times associated with forced swallowing. This suggests that the use of this maneuver should be avoided in patients who already have a delayed swallowing trigger time. The maneuver can be helpful in making pharyngeal clearance more efficient and prolonging the opening time of the upper esophageal sphincter. Forced swallowing can improve swallowing by increasing the forces applied to the bolus for its progression in the oropharyngeal channel. In the application of the maneuver, an important variable is the patient's ability to implement it. Monitoring the application of the maneuver may be useful, at least in the learning phases of biofeedback, for the electromyographic detection of muscle activity through surface electrodes. One study (Gomes et al. 2020) reported the onset of adverse events following the use of forced swallowing. The consecutive use of the forced swallowing maneuver for a period of 5 min caused cardiac overload in a young healthy woman. This effect has not been reported in other studies but suggests caution in the use of this forced swallowing maneuver in subjects with cardiac problems.

4.3.2 Decomposition of Swallowing

The conscious decomposition of swallowing into its individual phases allows the patient to become aware of each single phase of swallowing. Attention to each phase results in greater coordination and awareness of the swallowing mechanism. It is advisable to use the decomposition of swallowing in cases where postural compensation is used. In fact, very often, we assist patients who swallow before assuming the indicated position for the head, thus undermining the effects of posture. In these cases, a greater awareness of the swallowing mechanism helps with respect to the correct timing for the execution of the posture. In some subjects, the decomposition of swallowing can directly benefit swallowing functionality. In fact, sometimes the mere slowing down of swallowing can eliminate, or at least reduce, episodes of aspiration. Even with this maneuver, training induces an improvement in performance. A contraindication to the use of the decomposition of swallowing is the presence of cognitive deficits, which can determine poor patient compliance.

4.3.3 Supraglottic and Super-supraglottic Swallowing Maneuvers

The supraglottic and super-supraglottic swallowing maneuvers are techniques for protecting the airways from the passage of solid and liquid boluses through the closure of the airways before swallowing. Furthermore, in both maneuvers, at the end of the swallowing act, a cough is requested to clear the airways of any possible bolus residue. The difference between the two maneuvers lies in the effort required to achieve airway closure. In the super-supraglottic maneuver, greater effort is needed, whereas in the supraglottic maneuver, milder effort is needed. Both maneuvers are performed in four consecutive steps.

Supraglottic swallowing maneuver:

1. Take a deep breath.
2. Hold your breath.
3. Swallow.
4. Exhale by coughing.

Super-supraglottic swallowing maneuver:

1. Take a deep breath.
2. Forcefully hold your breath.
3. Swallow forcefully.
4. Exhale by coughing twice.

Closure of the vocal folds is one of the main mechanisms for protection of the lower airways (Shaker et al. 1990), so a technique that improves this closure increases the safety of the swallowing act, helping to reduce aspiration. The closure of the glottis was found to be complete only in 57–82% of a sample of healthy subjects who voluntarily held their breath (Mendelsohn and Martin 1993; Donzelli and Brady 2004). The degree of glottis closure increases in a situation of effort or in a phonatory situation (Mendelsohn and Martin 1993; Donzelli and Brady 2004; Martin et al. 1993). The visualization of the glottic closure with FEES reveals the difference in the glottic closure patterns in a normal situation of held breath and in a situation of forcefully held breath (Fig. 4.9).

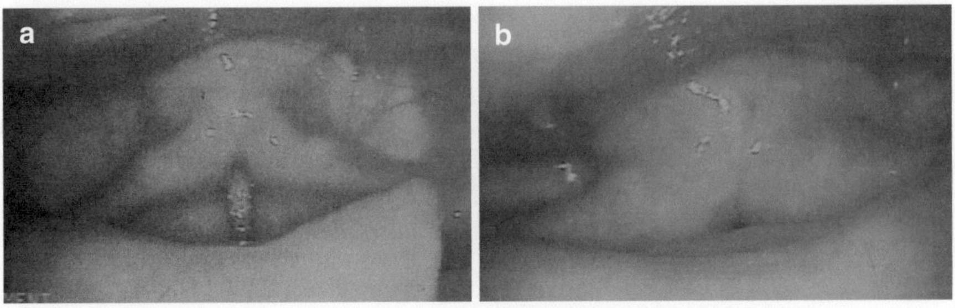

Fig. 4.9 Glottic closure: (**a**) during breath holding; (**b**) during forced breath holding

In forced closure, access to the lower airways is blocked not only by the approximation of the true vocal folds but also by the advancement of the arytenoids. Thus, it is closed in the two directions of horizontal and anterior closure. This closure pattern reproduces the normal closure pattern of the larynx during the swallowing act when, in the first phase, the vocal folds are approximated and, subsequently, during the vertical excursion of the larynx, the arytenoids move forward toward the base of the epiglottis. The maximum closure of the larynx, both horizontally and anteriorly, is reached at the highest point of laryngeal elevation (Flaherty et al. 1995). This type of closure is also achieved in the supraglottic swallowing maneuver and in the super-supraglottic maneuver. The execution of the maneuver presents a certain degree of difficulty because of the fixed sequence in which the various steps must be performed. This is difficult to overcome for subjects with cognitive impairment. There are many execution errors: one of the most frequent errors is when the patient begins breathing during the swallowing phase, thus impairing the benefits of the maneuver; in this case, endoscopic biofeedback proves to be a useful technique for teaching the maneuver. Another common error is made in the fourth step, when the patient, before exhaling by coughing, takes a breath: in this way, any pharyngeal residues are inevitably aspirated. Another aspect not to be overlooked is fatigue: the two maneuvers are in all respects compensations and therefore require constant commitment throughout the entire duration of the meal. Fatigue can reduce the accuracy of maneuver execution and cause cardiovascular effects in patients with heart disease or stroke (Chaudhuri et al. 2002).

4.3.4 Multiple Swallows

The consecutive repetition of two or more swallowing acts is also a strategy used by normal subjects to clear the oropharyngeal channel from any residue of boluses that is particularly difficult to swallow. In patients with dysphagia, it is a method often encouraged by the speech therapist, with the invitation to swallow again (Robbins et al. 1986; Dziadziola et al. 1992; Leslie et al. 2002). Various studies have reported its frequent use in healthy adults, mainly in older individuals (Nilsson et al. 1996), and during the swallowing of boluses with a particular taste (Pelletier and Lawless 2003). There is no strong evidence in the literature supporting or discouraging the clinical use of this maneuver. Multiple swallows can be a good technique during meals with reasonable caution. In fact, the use of multiple swallowing acts per bolus prolongs the duration of mealtime and causes fatigue in the patient: both elements can negatively contribute to caloric intake. It is preferable to perform the maneuver in a therapeutic program only after careful analysis of all the factors that could contraindicate its use.

4.3.5 Shaker Maneuver

The Shaker maneuver is a simple isometric and isotonic exercise that strengthens the suprahyoid muscles, reducing post-swallowing aspirations (Shaker et al. 1997, 2002), and can be performed both in the supine and sitting positions. In the supine position, the patient is asked to flex the head forward and look at the tips of the feet for 1 min; then, the head is extended and rested on the bed. The extension is maintained for 1 min, after which it returns to anterior flexion. Overall, the patient must alternately perform three flexions and three extensions, each lasting a minute, at the end of which he performs consecutively, in rapid succession, 30 flexion-extension movements of the head. The exercise can also be performed in a sitting position, in the *chin tuck against resistance* (CTAR) mode (Yoon et al. 2014), using a special spring that opposes resistance to the movement of the head. The exercise is performed in three daily training sessions for a period of 6 weeks (three times for 7 days for 6 weeks). The contraindications are related to the presence of problems of the cervical spine that discourage the repeated and forced flexion-extension of the head, the reduction of neck movements (present in some patients undergoing head-neck surgery), and the presence of a tracheostomy cannula or cognitive deficits that may determine the poor compliance of the patient with the daily training routine. Numerous studies have demonstrated the effectiveness of this maneuver: Shaker et al. (1997, 2002) have shown, in a sample of healthy adults, that the use of the maneuver increases the anterior excursion of the larynx, widens the opening times of the anterior esophageal sphincter, and reduces the number of post-swallowing aspirations. This effect did not occur in a similar sample of subjects who only performed generic exercises. In particular, the maneuver increases the strength of the suprahyoid muscles, which is considered the architect of the opening of the SES as a result of the elevation and anteriorization of the hyolaryngeal complex. Two studies (Ferdjallah et al. 2000; White et al. 2008) have demonstrated the activation of the supra- and infrahyoid muscles as a result of the execution of the Shaker maneuver. An example of the execution of the Shaker maneuver is available on the internet page https://www.mcw.edu/departments/medicine/divisions/gastroenterology-and-hepatology/patient-care/shaker-exercise.

4.3.6 Masako Maneuver

The Masako maneuver (Fujiu and Logemann 1996; Fujiu et al. 1995) is an exercise used in patients with reduced pharyngeal clearance due to insufficient lingual posteriorization and limited contraction of the pharynx. This maneuver induces forward movement of the posterior wall of the pharynx during swallowing, an effect observed for the first time in subjects undergoing surgical resection of 30% of the tongue. These patients, after a certain time from resection, showed swelling of the posterior wall of the pharynx that increased in proportion to the extent of resection. That is, patients with larger resection margins had greater swelling of the posterior wall of the pharynx. In other words, the anteriorization of the pharyngeal wall during swallowing somehow compensated for the reduction in the length of the tongue. The Masako maneuver is used to achieve the same result in subjects not undergoing tongue surgery. The exercise is performed by holding the tip of the tongue between the incisors. In this position, the patient performs dry swallows or repeats the syllable "ka." If the patient does not have incisors, an attempt is made to perform the exercise by holding the tip of the tongue between the lips. This method is more complex to perform because of the difficulty of holding the tongue with the lips alone. The Masako maneuver should not be used during meals (Fujiu and Logemann 1996) because it maintains its specificity in training to strengthen the posterior wall of the pharynx. In this way, the presence of residues in the pharynx is reduced (Lazarus et al. 2002).

4.3.7 Mendelsohn Maneuver

The Mendelsohn maneuver was developed to increase the vertical excursion of the larynx and consequently widen the opening of the upper esophageal sphincter. Specifically, the maneuver expands and prolongs the forward and upward excursion of the larynx and the hyoid bone, consequently increasing the degree of opening of the upper esophageal sphincter (Logemann 1988; Logemann and Kahrilas 1990). The maneuver also improves the coordination and timing of events during swallowing (Lazarus et al. 1993). One study (Ding et al. 2002) reported the strengthening of the suprahyoid and infrahyoid musculatures in a sample of healthy subjects as a result of the maneuver. Another study (Miller and Watkin 1997) reported an increase in the degree of medialization of the pharyngeal walls. The use of the maneuver has improved swallowing functionality in patients with postsurgical dysphagia and post-chemoradiotherapy treatment (Lazarus et al. 1993, 2002). The use of the Mendelsohn maneuver has also improved swallowing in patients with chronic stroke (Prosiegel et al. 2000; Robbins and Levine 1993; Huckabee and Cannito 1999). The maneuver is not very simple to perform and generally requires a training period during which the patient learns the correct method of execution to reproduce during training sessions. It involves the voluntary prolongation of the number of times the larynx is lifted. The patient trains to hold up the hyolaryngeal complex as long as possible, which normally lifts for a very short time while swallowing. To facilitate learning of the maneuver, the speech therapist may show on themselves the prolongation of the larynx elevation times during swallowing. When available, a biofeedback device can be used, both in the learning phase and for monitoring during training. By positioning the detection electrodes on the skin of the neck above the hyoid bone, it will be possible to highlight the prolonged activation of the musculature. Very useful in the learning phase are the use of a mirror and the promotion of self-palpation skills.

4.3.8 Rapid Mandibular Opening Maneuver

A rapid mandibular opening maneuver was recently proposed (Matsubara et al. 2018) with the aim of strengthening the suprahyoid musculature. The training of the suprahyoid musculature is important for the management of dysphagia and primarily aims to improve the insufficient opening of the upper esophageal sphincter during swallowing; as an exercise, the maneuver of rapid jaw opening should not be used during feeding. The exercise takes advantage of the opening of the jaw, as the suprahyoid muscles are equally involved in this movement, and the simple repeated opening of the jaw has proven to be an effective training for the suprahyoid musculature. In fact, a training scheme with isometric exercises of opening the jaw to the maximum degree for 10 s, with two sets of five repetitions per day for a period of 4 weeks, produced the result of raising the hyoid bone, raising the SES, improving its opening, and reducing the pharyngeal transit time (ibid.). This training method, however, does not involve fast-twitch muscle fibers, which make up more than half of the muscle fibers of the suprahyoid muscles and therefore are not involved in the execution of the isometric exercise of opening the jaw. A variant has therefore been introduced to the execution of the maneuver, with a high-speed jaw opening exercise aimed at stimulating the contraction of fast-twitch muscle fibers: the subject is invited to open the jaw to the maximum degree every 2 s, and each training set consists of 20 repetitions of rapid movement to the maximum degree of jaw opening.

In the execution of the exercise, the patient is assisted in maintaining the right rhythm via a metronome set at 30 beats per minute. The training scheme involves three sets of rapid jaw openings, each consisting of 20 repetitions interspersed with 10 s of rest, twice a day and for a period of 4 weeks. It is important to instruct subjects to feel the strong tension of the suprahyoid musculature during the opening of the jaw and to stop exercising if they notice any anomalies in the temporomandibular joint. The training program with the exercise of high-speed jaw opening produces a higher resting position of the hyoid bone in the neck, a greater degree of elevation during swallowing, and a wider degree of opening of the SES. The authors also reported a significant increase in the speed of elevation of the hyoid bone, which resulted in a reduction in the duration of the elevation itself and a reduction in the pharyngeal transit time. However, no significant improvement in the forward movement of the hyoid bone during swallowing was detected. The high-speed jaw opening exercise is useful for increasing the effectiveness of the fast-twitch fibers of the suprahyoid muscles.

4.4 Preventive Strategies

In recent years, a further preventive approach for dysphagic patients has been developed. Strictly speaking, even compensatory and rehabilitative approaches are preventive, as they prevent the onset of lung inflammation or the consequences resulting from insufficient nutritional intake. Strictly speaking, the preventive approach concerns preventing or minimizing the effects of dysphagia in patients undergoing chemoradiotherapy for head-neck district neoplasms. Interest in this type of approach has been increasing since the 2000s, with a significant increase in the last 6 years (Loewen et al. 2021). This development is justified by the fact that more than 80% of patients treated for oropharyngeal cancer show signs of dysphagia in daily life (Hutcheson et al. 2012). The increase in the survival of these patients emphasizes the long-term effects produced by radiotherapy treatments (Loewen et al. 2021). Moreover, the incidence of oropharyngeal tumors is increasing (Gillison et al. 2008; Stein et al. 2014). In the last 20 years, a worrying increase in the incidence of oropharyngeal tumors in young people has been reported: these neoplasms are not related to alcohol or tobacco consumption but rather to infection with the papillomavirus (human papillomavirus, HPV), the same agent responsible for cervical cancer, transmitted through the practice of oral sex (Stein et al. 2015). All these elements justify interest in the preventive approach, exemplified by prehabilitation. This consists of proactive training, that is, muscle training that includes protective elements capable of increasing resistance to stress of traumatic origin. In cancer patients, prehabilitation is a continuous care process that begins after diagnosis and, until acute treatment, provides specific interventions with the aim of reducing the incidence and severity of present or future impediments (Silver and Baima 2013). Historically, prehabilitation was introduced as a way to improve the nutritional and physical status of recruits enlisted in the army. In the field of health, it constitutes an opportunity capable of reducing hospitalization times and the related costs for health services. Prehabilitation has had its greatest use in orthopedics, such as the preparation of patients for the outcomes of surgical interventions. In oncology, impairments are addressed before they arise (Silver and Baima 2013; Silver et al. 2013, 2015). For several years, prehabilitation has also been used in the care of patients with head and neck tumors (Carroll et al. 2008; van der Molen et al. 2011). For this purpose, programs have been prepared that include specific exercises, of which the paradigm is defined, which consists of the number of repetitions for each step, the number of daily training sets, and the duration of such training. One of these is the UAB Dysphagia Protocol from the University of Alabama in Birmingham (UAB). The protocol includes five different exercises which the patient starts 2 weeks before chemoradiotherapy treatment and continues throughout the duration of the treatment:

1. The Masako maneuver
2. Tongue exercises against resistance
3. Forced swallowing
4. The Mendelsohn maneuver
5. Shaker exercises

Each exercise is repeated ten times in five different sessions distributed throughout the day. In each training session, the exercises are performed in a different sequence. In fact, it is inevitable that, especially during chemotherapy, when the patient has more difficulty performing them, the last exercises in the sequence are performed worse or in a reduced manner. Most studies report positive results following the use of treatment protocols prior to chemoradiotherapy (Kulbersh et al. 2006; Carroll et al. 2008; van der Molen et al. 2011; Kotz et al. 2012). Only one study reported the absence of improvements in a patient undergoing a preventive treatment protocol (Ahlberg et al. 2011). In general, the literature agrees in reporting a better quality of life in patients undergoing speech therapy pre-treatment than in those undergoing treatment exclusively post-chemoradiotherapy (Kulbersh et al. 2006).

References

Ahlberg A, Engström T, Nikolaidis P, Gunnarsson K, Johansson H, Sharp L, Laurell G. Early self-care rehabilitation of head and neck cancer patients. Acta Otolaryngol. 2011;131(5):552–61. https://doi.org/10.3109/00016489.2010.532157.

Albuquerque LCA, Pernambuco L, da Silva CM, Chateaubriand MM, da Silva HJ. Effects of electromyographic biofeedback as an adjunctive therapy in the treatment of swallowing disorders: a systematic review of the literature. Eur Arch Otorrinolaringol. 2019;276(4):927–38. https://doi.org/10.1007/s00405-019-05336-5.

American College of Sports Medicine. The recommended quantity and quality of exercise for developing and maintaining cardiorespiratory and muscular fitness, and flexibility in healthy adults. Med Sci Sports Exerc. 1998;30(6):975–91.

Ayuse T, Ayuse T, Ishitobi S, Kurata S, Sakamoto E, Okayasu I, Oi K. Effect of reclining and chin-tuck position on the coordination between respiration and swallowing. J Oral Rehabil. 2006;33(6):402–8. https://doi.org/10.1111/j.1365-2842.2005.01586.x.

Baijens LW, Speyer R, Roodenburg N, Manni JJ. The effects of neuromuscular electrical stimulation for dysphagia in opercular syndrome: a case study. Eur Arch Otorrinolaringol. 2008;265(7):825–30. https://doi.org/10.1007/s00405-007-0516-5.

Baijens LW, Speyer R, Passos VL, Pilz W, van der Kruis J, Haarmans S, Desjardins-Rombouts C. Surface electrical stimulation in dysphagic Parkinson patients: a randomized clinical trial. Laryngoscope. 2013;123(11):E38–44. https://doi.org/10.1002/lary.24119.

Barkmeier JM, Bielamowicz S, Takeda N, Ludlow CL. Laryngeal activity during upright vs. supine swallowing. J Appl Physiol. 2002;93(2):740–5. https://doi.org/10.1152/japplphysiol.00380.2001.

Bath PM, Scutt P, Love J, Clavé P, Cohen D, Dziewas R, Iversen HK, Ledl C, Ragab S, Soda H, Warusevitane A, Woisard V, Hamdy S, Swallowing Treatment Using Pharyngeal Electrical Stimulation (STEPS) Trial Investigators. Pharyngeal electrical stimulation for treatment of dysphagia in subacute stroke: a randomized controlled trial. Stroke. 2016;47(6):1562–70. https://doi.org/10.1161/STROKEAHA.115.012455.

Battel I, Calvo I, Walshe M. Interventions involving biofeedback to improve swallowing in people with Parkinson disease and dysphagia: a systematic review. Arch Phys Med Rehabil. 2021;102(2):314–22. https://doi.org/10.1016/j.apmr.2020.06.033.

Benfield JK, Everton LF, Bath PM, England TJ. Does therapy with biofeedback improve swallowing in adults with dysphagia? A systematic review and meta-analysis. Arch Phys Med Rehabil. 2019;100(3):551–61. https://doi.org/10.1016/j.apmr.2018.04.031.

Bhatt AD, Goodwin N, Cash E, Bhatt G, Silverman CL, Spanos WJ, Bumpous JM, Potts K, Redman R, Allison WA, Dunlap NE. Impact of transcutaneous neuromuscular electrical stimulation on dysphagia in patients with head and neck cancer treated with definitive chemoradiation. Head Neck. 2015;37(7):1051–6. https://doi.org/10.1002/hed.23708.

Blumenfeld L, Hahn Y, Lepage A, Leonard R, Belafsky PC. Transcutaneous electrical stimulation versus traditional dysphagia therapy: a nonconcurrent cohort study. Otolaryngol Head Neck Surg. 2006;135(5):754–7. https://doi.org/10.1016/j.otohns.2006.04.016.

Bülow M, Olsson R, Ekberg O. Videomanometric analysis of Supraglottic swallow, effortful swallow, and Chin Tuck in healthy volunteers. Dysphagia. 1999;14(2):67–72.

Bülow M, Olsson R, Ekberg O. Videomanometric analysis of supraglottic swallow, effortful swallow, and chin tuck in patients with pharyngeal dysfunction. Dysphagia. 2001;16(3):190–5. https://doi.org/10.1007/s00455-001-0065-9.

Bülow M, Olsson R, Ekberg O. Videoradiographic analysis of how carbonated thin liquids and thickened liquids affect the physiology of swallowing in subjects with aspiration on thin liquids. Acta Radiol. 2003;44(4):366–72. https://doi.org/10.1080/j.1600-0455.2003.00100.x.

Bülow M, Speyer R, Baijens L, Woisard V, Ekberg O. Neuromuscular electrical stimulation (NMES) in stroke patients with oral and pharyngeal dysfunction. Dysphagia. 2008;23(3):302–9. https://doi.org/10.1007/s00455-007-9145-9.

Campbell G, Shatz CJ. Synapses formed by identified retinogeniculate axons during the segregation of eye input. J Neurosci. 1992;12(5):1847–58. https://doi.org/10.1523/JNEUROSCI.12-05-01847.

Carey JR, Kimberley TJ, Lewis SM, Auerbach EJ, Dorsey L, Rundquist P, Ugurbil K. Analysis of fMRI and finger tracking training in subjects with chronic stroke. Brain. 2002;125(Pt 4):773–88. https://doi.org/10.1093/brain/awf091.

Carnaby-Mann GD, Crary MA. Adjunctive neuromuscular electrical stimulation for treatment-refractory dysphagia. Ann Otol Rhinol Laryngol. 2008;117(4):279–87. https://doi.org/10.1177/000348940811700407.

Carnaby-Mann GD, Crary MA. McNeill dysphagia therapy program: a case-control study. Arch Phys Med Rehabil. 2010;91(5):743–9. https://doi.org/10.1016/j.apmr.2010.01.013.

Carnaby-Mann G, et al. A randomized double blind trial of neuromuscular electrical stimulation + McNeill Dysphagia Therapy (MDTP) after Stroke (ANSRS). Presented at Dysphagia Research Society, Toronto, Canada, March 7–10; 2012.

Carroll WR, Locher JL, Canon CL, Bohannon IA, McColloch NL, Magnuson JS. Pretreatment swallowing exercises improve swallow function after chemoradiation. Laryngoscope. 2008;118(1):39–43. https://doi.org/10.1097/MLG.0b013e31815659b0.

Castell JA, Dalton CB, Castell DO. Effects of body position and bolus consistency on the manometric parameters and coordination of the upper esophageal sphincter and pharynx. Dysphagia. 1990;5(4):179–86. https://doi.org/10.1007/BF02412685.

Castell JA, Castell DO, Schultz AR, Georgeson S. Effect of head position on the dynamics of the upper esophageal sphincter and pharynx. Dysphagia. 1993;8(1):1–6. https://doi.org/10.1007/BF01351470.

Chaudhuri G, Hildner CD, Brady S, Hutchins B, Aliga N, Abadilla E. Cardiovascular effects of the supraglottic and super-supraglottic swallowing maneuvers in stroke patients with dysphagia. Dysphagia. 2002;17(1):19–23. https://doi.org/10.1007/s00455-001-0097-1.

Chee C, Arshad S, Singh S, Mistry S, Hamdy S. The influence of chemical gustatory stimuli and oral anaesthesia on healthy human pharyngeal swallowing. Chem Senses. 2005;30(5):393–400. https://doi.org/10.1093/chemse/bji034.

Cichero JAY, Murdoch BE. Dysphagia: foundation, theory and practice. Brisbane: Wiley; 2006.

Cichero JA, Jackson O, Halley PJ, Murdoch BE. How thick is thick? Multicenter study of the rheological and material property characteristics of mealtime fluids and videofluoroscopy fluids. Dysphagia. 2000;15(4):188–200. https://doi.org/10.1007/s004550000027.

Clark HM. Neuromuscular treatments for speech and swallowing: a tutorial. Am J Speech Lang Pathol. 2003;12(4):400–15.

Clark HM, O'Brien K, Calleja A, Corrie SN. Effects of directional exercise on lingual strength. J Speech Lang Hear Res. 2009;52(4):1034–47. https://doi.org/10.1044/1092-4388(2009/08-0062).

Coyle JL. Water, water everywhere, but why?Argument against free water protocols. Perspect ASHA Spec Interest Groups. 2011;20(4):109–15.

Crary MA, Groher ME. Basic concepts of surface electromyographic biofeedback in the treatment of dysphagia: a tutorial. Am J Speech Lang Pathol. 2000;9(2):116–25.

Crary MA, Groher ME. Reinstituting oral feeding in tube-fed adult patients with dysphagia. Nutr Clin Pract. 2006;21(6):576–86.
Daniels SK, Huckabee ML. Dysphagia following stroke. San Diego/Oxford: Plural Pub; 2008.
Ding R, Larson CR, Logemann JA, Rademaker AW. Surface electromyographic and electroglottographic studies in normal subjects under two swallow conditions: normal and during the Mendelsohn manuever. Dysphagia. 2002;17(1):1–12. https://doi.org/10.1007/s00455-001-0095-3.
Donzelli J, Brady S. The effects of breath-holding on vocal fold adduction: implications for safe swallowing. Arch Otolaryngol-Head Neck Surg. 2004;130(2):208–10.
Duchateau J, Hainaut K. Isometric or dynamic training: differential effects on mechanical properties of a human muscle. J Appl Physiol Respir Environ Exerc Physiol. 1984;56(2):296–301.
Dysphagia Team of Seirei, Fujishima I. Pocket manual of dysphagia. 3rd ed. Tokyo: Ishiyaku Publications; 2011.
Dziadziola J, Hamlet S, Michou G, Jones L. Multiple swallows and piecemeal deglutition; observations from normal adults and patients with head and neck cancer. Dysphagia. 1992;7(1):8–11. https://doi.org/10.1007/BF02493415.
Dziewas R, Stellato R, van der Tweel I, Walther E, Werner CJ, Braun T, Citerio G, Jandl M, Friedrichs M, Nötzel K, Vosko MR, Mistry S, Hamdy S, McGowan S, Warnecke T, Zwittag P, Bath PM, PHAST-TRAC investigators. Pharyngeal electrical stimulation for early decannulation in tracheotomised patients with neurogenic dysphagia after stroke (PHAST-TRAC): a prospective, single-blinded, randomised trial. Lancet Neurol. 2018;17(10):849–59. https://doi.org/10.1016/S1474-4422(18)30255-2.
Ekberg O. Posture of the head and pharyngeal swallowing. Acta Radiol Diagn. 1986;27(6):691–6.
El Sharkawi A, Ramig L, Logemann JA, Pauloski BR, Rademaker AW, Smith CH, Pawlas A, Baum S, Werner C. Swallowing and voice effects of Lee Silverman Voice Treatment (LSVT): a pilot study. J Neurol Neurosurg Psychiatry. 2002;72(1):31–6. https://doi.org/10.1136/jnnp.72.1.31.
Elbert T, Heim S. A light and a dark side. Nature. 2001;411(6834):139.
Feinberg MJ, Knebl J, Tully J, Segall L. Aspiration and the elderly. Dysphagia. 1990;5(2):61–71. https://doi.org/10.1007/BF02412646.
Feinberg MJ, Knebl J, Tully J. Prandial aspiration and pneumoniain an elderly population followed over 3 years. Dysphagia. 1996;11(2):104–9.
Ferdjallah M, Wertsch JJ, Shaker R. Spectral analysis of surface electromyography (EMG) of upper esophageal sphincter-opening muscles during head lift exercise. J Rehabil Res Dev. 2000;37(3):335–40.
Fiatarone MA, Marks EC, Ryan ND, Meredith CN, Lipsitz LA, Evans WJ. High-intensity strength training in nonagenarians. Effects on skeletal muscle. JAMA. 1990;263(22):3029–34.
Flaherty RF, Seltzer S, Campbell T, Weisskoff RM, Gilbert RJ. Dynamic magnetic resonance imaging of vocal cord closure during deglutition. Gastroenterology. 1995;109(3):843–9. https://doi.org/10.1016/0016-5085(95)90393-3.
Freed ML, Freed L, Chatburn RL, Christian M. Electrical stimulation for swallowing disorders caused by stroke. Respir Care. 2001;46(5):466–74.
Fujiu M, Logemann JA. Effect of a tongue-holding maneuver on posterior pharyngeal wall movement during deglutition. Am J Speech Lang Pathol. 1996;5(1):23–30.
Fujiu M, Logemann JA, Pauloski B. Increased postoperative posterior pharyngeal wall movement in patients with anterior oral cancer preliminary findings and possible implications for treatment. Am J Speech Lang Pathol. 1995;4(2):24–30.
Gaita A, et al. The dysphagic patient: manual for relatives and caregivers. In: ISTISAN reports, 08/38. Rome: Higher Institute of Health; 2008. http://www.airas.it/wpcontent/uploads/20u/04/dysphagia_advice_to_relatives.pdf.
Garcia JM, Chambers E 4th, Molander M. Thickened liquids: practice patterns of speech-language pathologists. Am J Speech Lang Pathol. 2005;14(1):4–13. https://doi.org/10.1044/1058-0360(2005/003).

Giggins OM, Persson UM, Caulfield B. Biofeedback in rehabilitation. J Neuroeng Rehabil. 2013;10:60. https://doi.org/10.1186/1743-0003-10-60.

Gillison ML, D'Souza G, Westra W, Sugar E, Xiao W, Begum S, Viscidi R. Distinct risk factor profiles for human papillomavirus type 16-positive and human papillomavirus type 16-negative head and neck cancers. J Natl Cancer Inst. 2008;100(6):407–20. https://doi.org/10.1093/jnci/djn025.

Gillman A, Winkler R, Taylor NF. Implementing the free water protocol does not result in aspiration pneumonia in carefully selected patients with dysphagia: a systematic review. Dysphagia. 2017;32(3):345–61. https://doi.org/10.1007/s00455-016-9761-3.

Gomes LMS, da Silva RG, Pedroni CR, Garner DM, Raimundo RD, Valenti VE. Effects of effortful swallowing on cardiac autonomic control in individuals with neurogenic dysphagia: a prospective observational analytical study. Sci Rep. 2020;10:10924.

Groher ME, Crary MA. Dysphagia. St. Louis: Elsevier; 2021.

Hiss SG, Huckabee ML. Timing of pharyngeal and upper esophageal sphincter pressures as a function of normal and effortful swallowing in young healthy adults. Dysphagia. 2005;20(2):149–56.

Holas MA, DePippo KL, Reding MJ. Aspiration and relative risk of medical complications following stroke. Arch Neurol. 1994;51(10):1051–3.

Huckabee ML, Cannito MP. Outcomes of swallowing rehabilitation in chronic brainstem dysphagia: a retrospective evaluation. Dysphagia. 1999;14(2):93–109.

Huckabee ML, Butler SG, Barclay M, Jit S. Submental surface electromyographic measurement and pharyngeal pressures during normal and effortful swallowing. Arch Phys Med Rehabil. 2005;86(11):2144–9. https://doi.org/10.1016/j.apmr.2005.05.005.

Humbert IA, German RZ. New directions for understanding neural control in swallowing: the potential and promise of motor learning. Dysphagia. 2013;28(1):1–10.

Hutcheson KA, Lewin JS, Barringer DA, Lisec A, Gunn GB, Moore MW, Holsinger FC. Late dysphagia after radiotherapy-based treatment of head and neck cancer. Cancer. 2012;118(23):5793–9. https://doi.org/10.1002/cncr.27631.

Hutcheson KA, Barrow MP, Plowman EK, Lai SY, Fuller CD, Barringer DA, Eapen G, Wang Y, Hubbard R, Jimenez SK, Little LG, Lewin JS. Expiratory muscle strength training for radiation-associated aspiration after head and neck cancer: a case series. Laryngoscope. 2018;128(5):1044–51. https://doi.org/10.1002/lary.26845.

Ingervall B, Lantz B. Significance of gravity on the passage of bolus through the human pharynx. Arch Oral Biol. 1973;18(3):351–6.

Jayasekeran V, Singh S, Tyrrell P, Michou E, Jefferson S, Mistry S, Gamble E, Rothwell J, Thompson D, Hamdy S. Adjunctive functional pharyngeal electrical stimulation reverses swallowing disability after brain lesions. Gastroenterology. 2010;138(5):1737–46. https://doi.org/10.1053/j.gastro.2010.01.052.

Kandel E, et al. Principles of neuroscience. In: Perri V, Spidalieri G, editors. . Milan: Casa Editrice Ambrosiana; 2014.

Karagiannis M, Karagiannis TC. Oropharyngeal dysphagia, free water protocol and quality of life: an update from a prospective clinical trial. Hell J Nucl Med. 2014;17(Suppl 1):26–9.

Kiger M, Brown CS, Watkins L. Dysphagia management: an analysis of patient outcomes using VitalStim therapy compared to traditional swallow therapy. Dysphagia. 2006;21(4):243–53. https://doi.org/10.1007/s00455-006-9056-1.

Kilgard MP, Merzenich MM. Cortical map reorganization enabled by nucleus basalis activity. Science. 1998;279(5357):1714–8. https://doi.org/10.1126/science.279.5357.

Kim CK, Ryu JS, Song SH, Koo JH, Lee KD, Park HS, Oh Y, Min K. Effects of head rotation and head tilt on pharyngeal pressure events using high resolution manometry. Ann Rehabil Med. 2015;39(3):425–31. https://doi.org/10.5535/arm.2015.39.3.425.

Kirchner JA. Pharyngeal and esophageal dysfunction: the diagnosis. Minn Med. 1967;50(6):921–4.

Kleim JA, Jones TA. Principles of experience-dependent neural plasticity: implication for rehabilitation after brain damage. J Speech Lang Hearing Res. 2008;51(1):225–39.

Kolb B, Gibb R. Searching for the principles of brain plasticity and behavior. Cortex. 2014;58:251–60.

Kotz T, Federman AD, Kao J, Milman L, Packer S, Lopez-Prieto C, Forsythe K, Genden EM. Prophylactic swallowing exercises in patients with head and neck cancer undergoing chemoradiation: a randomized trial. Arch Otolaryngol Head Neck Surg. 2012;138(4):376–82. https://doi.org/10.1001/archoto.2012.187.

Krakauer JW. Motor learning: its relevance to stroke recovery and neurorehabilitation. Curr Opin Neurol. 2006;19(1):84–90.

Krival K, Bates C. Effects of club soda and ginger brew on linguapalatal pressures in healthy swallowing. Dysphagia. 2012;27(2):228–39.

Kuhlemeier KV, Palmer JB, Rosenberg D. Effect of liquid bolus consistency and delivery method on aspiration and pharyngeal retention in dysphagia patients. Dysphagia. 2001;16(2):119–22.

Kulbersh BD, Rosenthal EL, McGrew BM, Duncan RD, McColloch NL, Carroll WR, Magnuson JS. Pretreatment, preoperative swallowing exercises may improve dysphagia quality of life. Laryngoscope. 2006;116(6):883–6. https://doi.org/10.1097/01.mlg.0000217278.96901.fc.

Kushner DS, Peters K, Eroglu ST, Perless-Carroll M, Johnson-Greene D. Neuromuscular electrical stimulation efficacy in acute stroke feeding tube-dependent dysphagia during inpatient rehabilitation. Am J Phys Med Rehabil. 2013;92(6):486–95. https://doi.org/10.1097/PHM.0b013e31828762ec.

Langmore SE. Endoscopic evaluation and treatment of swallowing disorders. 2nd ed. New York: Thieme; 2001.

Langmore SE. Why I like the free water protocol. Perspect ASHA Spec Interest Groups. 2011;20(4):H6–20.

Larsson V, Torisson G, Bülow M, Londos E. Effects of carbonated liquid on swallowing dysfunction in dementia with Lewy bodies and Parkinson's disease dementia. Clin Interv Aging. 2017;12:1215–22. https://doi.org/10.2147/CIA.S140389.

Lazarus C, Logemann JA, Gibbons P. Effects of maneuvers on swallowing function in a dysphagic oral cancer patient. Head Neck. 1993;15(5):419–24.

Lazarus C, Logemann JA, Song CW, Rademaker AW, Kahrilas PJ. Effects of voluntary maneuvers on tongue base function for swallowing. Folia Phoniatr Logop. 2002;54(4):171–6. https://doi.org/10.1159/000063192.

Lazarus C, Logemann JA, Huang CF, Rademaker AW. Effects of two types of tongue strengthening exercises in young normals. Folia Phoniatr Logop. 2003;55(4):199–205. https://doi.org/10.1159/000071019.

Leelamanit V, Limsakul C, Geater A. Synchronized electrical stimulation in treating pharyngeal dysphagia. Laryngoscope. 2002;112(12):2204–10. https://doi.org/10.1097/00005537-200212000-00015.

Leslie P, Drinnan MJ, Ford GA, Wilson JA. Swallow respiration patterns in dysphagic patients following acute stroke. Dysphagia. 2002;17(3):202–7. https://doi.org/10.1007/s00455-002-0053-8.

Lewin JS, Hebert TM, Putnam JB Jr, DuBrow RA. Experience with the chin tuck maneuver in postesophagectomy aspirators. Dysphagia. 2001;16(3):216–9. https://doi.org/10.1007/s00455-001-0068-6.

Loewen I, Jeffery CC, Rieger J, Constantinescu G. Prehabilitation in head and neck cancer patients: a literature review. J Otolaryngol Head Neck Surg. 2021;50(1):2. https://doi.org/10.1186/s40463-020-00486-7.

Logemann JA. Swallowing physiology and pathophysiology. Otolaryngol Clin N Am. 1988;21(4):613–23.

Logemann JA. Behavioural management for oropharyngeal dysphagia. Folia Phoniatr Logop. 1999;51(4–5):199–213.

Logemann JA, Kahrilas PJ. Relearning to swallow after stroke-application of maneuvers and indirect biofeedback: a case study. Neurology. 1990;40(7):1136–8.

Logemann JA, Kahrilas PJ, Kobara M, Vakil NB. The benefit of head rotation on pharyngoesophageal dysphagia. Arch Phys Med Rehabil. 1989;70(10):767–71.

Logemann JA, Rademaker AW, Pauloski BR, Kahrilas PJ. Effects of postural change on aspiration in head and neck surgical patients. Otolaryngol Head Neck Surg. 1994;110(2):222–7. https://doi.org/10.1177/019459989411000212.

Logemann JA, Gensler G, Robbins J, Lindblad AS, Brandt D, Hind JA, Kosek S, Dikeman K, Kazandjian M, Gramigna GD, Lundy D, McGarvey-Toler S, Miller Gardner PJ. A randomized study of three interventions for aspiration of thin liquids in patients with dementia or Parkinson's disease. J Speech Lang Hear Res. 2008;51(1):173–83. https://doi.org/10.1044/1092-4388(2008/013).

Maas E, Robin DA, Austermann Hula SN, Freedman SE, Wulf G, Ballard KJ, Schmidt RA. Principles of motor learning in treatment of motor speech disorders. Am J Speech Lang Pathol. 2008;17(3):277–98. https://doi.org/10.1044/1058-0360(2008/025).

Malandraki GA, Rajappa A, Kantarcigil C, Wagner E, Ivey C, Youse K. The intensive dysphagia rehabilitation approach applied to patients with neurogenic dysphagia: a case series design study. Arch Phys Med Rehabil. 2016;97(4):567–74. https://doi.org/10.1016/j.apmr.2015.11.019.

Martin RE. Neuroplasticity and swallowing. Dysphagia. 2009;24(2):218–29.

Martin BJ, Logemann JA, Shaker R, Dodds WJ. Normal laryngeal valving patterns during three breath-hold maneuvers: a pilot investigation. Dysphagia. 1993;8(1):11–20. https://doi.org/10.1007/BF01351472.

Matsubara M, Tohara H, Hara K, Shinozaki H, Yamazaki Y, Susa C, Nakane A, Wakasugi Y, Minakuchi S. High-speed jaw-opening exercise in training suprahyoid fast-twitch muscle fibers. Clin Interv Aging. 2018;13:125–31. https://doi.org/10.2147/CIA.S152821.

McCauley RJ, Strand E, Lof GL, Schooling T, Frymark T. Evidence-based systematic review: effects of nonspeech oral motor exercises on speech. Am J Speech Lang Pathol. 2009;18(4):343–60. https://doi.org/10.1044/1058-0360(2009/09-0006).

McCulloch TM, Hoffman MR, Ciucci MR. High-resolution manometry of pharyngeal swallow pressure events associated with head turn and chin tuck. Ann Otol Rhinol Laryngol. 2010;119(6):369–76. https://doi.org/10.1177/000348941011900602.

Mendelsohn MS, Martin RE. Airway protection during breath-holding. Ann Otol Rhinol Laryngol. 1993;102(12):941–4.

Miller JL, Watkin KL. Lateral pharyngeal wall motion during swallowing using real time ultrasound. Dysphagia. 1997;12(3):125–32.

Miyaoka Y, Haishima K, Takagi M, Haishima H, Asari J, Yamada Y. Influences of thermal and gustatory characteristics on sensory and motor aspects of swallowing. Dysphagia. 2006;21(1):38–48. https://doi.org/10.1007/s00455-005-9003-6.

Mulder T, Hulstyn W. Sensory feedback therapy and theoretical knowledge of motor control and learning. Am J Phys Med. 1984;63(5):226–44.

Murray J, Langmore SE, Ginsberg S, Dostie A. The significance of accumulated oropharyngeal secretions and swallowing frequency in predicting aspiration. Dysphagia. 1996;11(2):99–103. https://doi.org/10.1007/BF00417898.

Nagy A, Peladeau-Pigeon M, Valenzano TJ, Namasivayam AM, Steele CM. The effectiveness of the head-turn-plus-chin-down maneuver for eliminating vallecular residue. Codas. 2016;28(2):113–7. https://doi.org/10.1590/2317-1782/20162015286.

National Dysphagia Diet Task Force. The National Dysphagia Diet: standardization for optimal care. Chicago: American Dietetic Association; 2002.

Nilsson H, Ekberg O, Olsson R, Hindfelt B. Quantitative aspects of swallowing in an elderly nondysphagic population. Dysphagia. 1996;11(3):180–4. https://doi.org/10.1007/BF00366381.

Nudo RJ, Wise BM, SiFuentes F, Milliken GW. Neural substrates for the effects of rehabilitative training on motor recovery after ischemic infarct. Science. 1996;272(5269):1791–4. https://doi.org/10.1126/science.272.5269.1791.

O'Gara JA. Dietary adjustments and nutritional therapy during treatment for oral-pharyngeal dysphagia. Dysphagia. 1990;4(4):209–12.

Oh BM, Kim DY, Paik NJ. Recovery of swallowing function is accompanied by the expansion of the cortical map. Int J Neurosci. 2007;117(9):1215–27.

Olson M. The benign effects on rabbits' lungs of the aspiration of water compared with 5 per cent glucose or milk. Pediatrics. 1970;46(4):538–47.

Palmer PM, Jaffe DM, McCulloch TM, Finnegan EM, Van Daele DJ, Luschei ES. Quantitative contributions of the muscles of the tongue, floor-of-mouth, jaw, and velum to tongue-to-palate pressure generation. J Speech Lang Hear Res. 2008;51(4):828–35. https://doi.org/10.1044/1092-4388(2008/060).

Panther K. The Frazier free water protocol: safety, hydration, and quality of life. Rockville: American Speech-Language-Hearing Association; 2008.

Pardoe EM. Development of a multistage diet for dysphagia. J Am Diet Assoc. 1993;93(5):568–71.

Pascual-Leone A, Amedi A, Fregni F, Merabet LB. The plastic human brain cortex. Annu Rev Neurosci. 2005;28:377–401. https://doi.org/10.1146/annurev.neuro.27.070203.144216.

Pelletier CA, Lawless HT. Effect of citric acid and citric acid-sucrose mixtures on swallowing in neurogenic oropharyngeal dysphagia. Dysphagia. 2003;18(4):231–41.

Pisegna J, Langmore S. The ice chip protocol: a description of the protocol and case reports. Perspect ASHA Spec Interest Groups. 2018;3(13):28–46.

Portale G, Peters J, Hsieh CC, Tamhankar A, Arain M, Hagen J, DeMeester S, DeMeester T. When are reflux episodes symptomatic? Dis Esophagus. 2007;20(1):47–52. https://doi.org/10.1111/j.1442-2050.2007.00650.x.

Powers S, Howley E. Exercise physiology. Theory and application to fitness and performance. New York: McGraw-Hill; 2008.

Prosiegel M, Heintze M, Sonntag EW, Schenk T, Yassouridis A. Kinematic analysis of laryngeal movements in patients with neurogenic dysphagia before and after swallowing rehabilitation. Dysphagia. 2000;15(4):173–9. https://doi.org/10.1007/s004550000024.

Reimers-Neils L, Logemann J, Larson C. Viscosity effects on EMG activity in normal swallowing. Dysphagia. 1994;9(2):101–6.

Restivo D, Hamdy S. Pharyngeal electrical stimulation device for the treatment of neurogenic dysphagia: technology update. Med Devices. 2018;11:21–6.

Robbins J, Levine R. Swallowing after lateral medullary syndrome plus. Clin Commun Disorder. 1993;3(4):45–55.

Robbins JA, Logemann JA, Kirshner HS. Swallowing and speech production in Parkinson's disease. Ann Neurol. 1986;19(3):283–7.

Robbins J, Gangnon RE, Theis SM, Kays SA, Hewitt AL, Hind JA. The effects of lingual exercise on swallowing in older adults. J Am Geriatr Soc. 2005;53(9):1483–9. https://doi.org/10.1111/j.1532-5415.2005.53467.x.

Robbins J, Kays SA, Gangnon RE, Hind JA, Hewitt AL, Gentry LR, Taylor AJ. The effects of lingual exercise in stroke patients with dysphagia. Arch Phys Med Rehabil. 2007;88(2):150–8. https://doi.org/10.1016/j.apmr.2006.11.002.

Robbins J, Gensler G, Hind J, Logemann JA, Lindblad AS, Brandt D, Baum H, Lilienfeld D, Kosek S, Lundy D, Dikeman K, Kazandjian M, Gramigna GD, McGarvey-Toler S, Miller Gardner PJ. Comparison of 2 interventions for liquid aspiration on pneumonia incidence: a randomized trial. Ann Intern Med. 2008;148(7):509–18. https://doi.org/10.7326/0003-4819-148-7-200804010-00007.

Ryu JS, Kang JY, Park JY, Nam SY, Choi SH, Roh JL, Kim SY, Choi KH. The effect of electrical stimulation therapy on dysphagia following treatment for head and neck cancer. Oral Oncol. 2009;45(8):665–8. https://doi.org/10.1016/j.oraloncology.2008.10.005.

Schindler O. Manual of pathophysiology of swallowing. Turin: Omega Editions; 1990.

Schindler O, Ruoppolo G, Schindler A. Deglutology. Turin: Omega Editions; 2011.

Schindler A, Pizzorni N, Cereda E, Cosentino G, Avenali M, Montomoli C, Abbruzzese G, Antonini A, Barbiera F, Benazzo M, Benarroch E, Bertino G, Clavè P, Cortelli P, Eleopra R, Ferrari C, Hamdy S, Huckabee ML, Lopiano L, Marchese-Ragona R, Masiero S, Michou E, Occhini A, Pacchetti C, Pfeiffer RF, Restivo DA, Rondanelli M, Ruoppolo G, Sandrini G, Schapira A, Stocchi F, Tolosa E, Valentino F, Zamboni M, Zangaglia R, Zappia M, Tassorelli C, Alfonsi E. Consensus on the treatment of dysphagia in Parkinson's disease. J Neurol Sci. 2021;430:120008. https://doi.org/10.1016/j.jns.2021.120008.

Scibilia S, Hreha K, Piscopo C, Adler U, Barrett AM. Implementing a free water protocol in an inpatient rehabilitation facility: outcomes and care transitions. Arch Phys Med Rehabil. 2016;97(10):e77.

Scutt P, Lee HS, Hamdy S, Bath PM. Pharyngeal electrical stimulation for treatment of poststroke dysphagia: individual patient data meta-analysis of randomised controlled trials. Stroke Res Treat. 2015;2015:429053. https://doi.org/10.1155/2015/429053.

Shaker R, Dodds WJ, Dantas RO, Hogan WJ, Arndorfer RC. Coordination of deglutitive glottic closure with oropharyngeal swallowing. Gastroenterology. 1990;98(6):1478–84. https://doi.org/10.1016/0016-5085(90)91078-k.

Shaker R, Kern M, Bardan E, Taylor A, Stewart ET, Hoffmann RG, Arndorfer RC, Hofmann C, Bonnevier J. Augmentation of deglutitive upper esophageal sphincter opening in the elderly by exercise. Am J Phys. 1997;272(6 Pt 1):G1518–22. https://doi.org/10.1152/ajpgi.1997.272.6.G1518.

Shaker R, Easterling C, Kern M, Nitschke T, Massey B, Daniels S, Grande B, Kazandjian M, Dikeman K. Rehabilitation of swallowing by exercise in tube-fed patients with pharyngeal dysphagia secondary to abnormal UES opening. Gastroenterology. 2002;122(5):1314–21. https://doi.org/10.1053/gast.2002.32999.

Shanahan TK, Logemann JA, Rademaker AW, Pauloski BR, Kahrilas PJ. Chin-down posture effect on aspiration in dysphagic patients. Arch Phys Med Rehabil. 1993;74(7):736–9. https://doi.org/10.1016/0003-9993(93)90035-9.

Shaw C, McEachern J. Toward a theory of neuroplasticity. Hove: Psychology Press; 2001.

Shaw GY, Sechtem PR, Searl J, Keller K, Rawi TA, Dowdy E. Transcutaneous neuromuscular electrical stimulation (VitalStim) curative therapy for severe dysphagia: myth or reality? Ann Otol Rhinol Laryngol. 2007;116(1):36–44. https://doi.org/10.1177/000348940711600107.

Shim JS, Oh BM, Han TR. Factors associated with compliance with viscosity-modified diet among dysphagic patients. Ann Rehabil Med. 2013;37(5):628–32. https://doi.org/10.5535/arm.2013.37.5.628.

Silver JK, Baima J. Cancer prehabilitation: an opportunity to decrease treatment-related morbidity, increase cancer treatment options, and improve physical and psychological health outcomes. Am J Phys Med Rehabil. 2013;92(8):715–27. https://doi.org/10.1097/PHM.0b013e31829b4afe.

Silver JK, Baima J, Mayer RS. Impairment-driven cancer rehabilitation: an essential component of quality care and survivorship. CA A Cancer J Clin. 2013;63(5):295–317.

Silver JK, Raj VS, Fu JB, Wisotzky EM, Smith SR, Kirch RA. Cancer rehabilitation and palliative care: critical components in the delivery of high-quality oncology services. Support Care Cancer. 2015;23(12):3633–43. https://doi.org/10.1007/s00520-015-2916-1.

Simonelli M, Ruoppolo G, de Vincentiis M, Di Mario M, Calcagno P, Vitiello C, Manciocco V, Pagliuca G, Gallo A. Swallowing ability and chronic aspiration after supracricoid partial laryngectomy. Otolaryngol Head Neck Surg. 2010;142(6):873–8. https://doi.org/10.1016/j.otohns.2010.01.035.

Splaingard ML, Hutchins B, Sulton LD, Chaudhuri G. Aspiration in rehabilitation patients: videofluoroscopy vs bedside clinical assessment. Arch Phys Med Rehabil. 1988;69(8):637–40.

Stein AP, Saha S, Yu M, Kimple RJ, Lambert PF. Prevalence of human papillomavirus in oropharyngeal squamous cell carcinoma in the United States across time. Chem Res Toxicol. 2014;27(4):462–9. https://doi.org/10.1021/tx500034c.

Stein AP, Saha S, Kraninger JL, Swick AD, Yu M, Lambert PF, Kimple RJ. Prevalence of human papillomavirus in oropharyngeal cancer: a systematic review. Cancer J. 2015;21(3):138–46. https://doi.org/10.1097/PPO.0000000000000115.

Suntrup S, Marian T, Schröder JB, Suttrup I, Muhle P, Oelenberg S, Hamacher C, Minnerup J, Warnecke T, Dziewas R. Electrical pharyngeal stimulation for dysphagia treatment in tracheotomized stroke patients: a randomized controlled trial. Intensive Care Med. 2015;41(9):1629–37. https://doi.org/10.1007/s00134-015-3897-8.

Takeishi R, Magara J, Watanabe M, Tsujimura T, Hayashi H, Hori K, Inoue M. Effects of pharyngeal electrical stimulation on swallowing performance. PLoS One. 2018;13(1):e0190608. https://doi.org/10.1371/journal.pone.0190608.

Tan C, Liu Y, Li W, Liu J, Chen L. Transcutaneous neuromuscular electrical stimulation can improve swallowing function in patients with dysphagia caused by non-stroke diseases: a meta-analysis. J Oral Rehabil. 2013;40(6):472–80. https://doi.org/10.1111/joor.12057.

Temple M, O'Leary D, Faden A. The role of glutamate receptors in the pathophysiology of traumatic CNS injury. In: Miller L, Hayes R, editors. Head trauma. Basic, preclinical and clinical directions. New York: Wiley; 2001. p. 87–113.

Terré R, Mearin F. Effectiveness of chin-down posture to prevent tracheal aspiration in dysphagia secondary to acquired brain injury. A videofluoroscopy study. Neurogastroenterol Motil. 2012;24(5):414–9, e206. https://doi.org/10.1111/j.1365-2982.2011.01869.x.

Troche MS, Okun MS, Rosenbek JC, Musson N, Fernandez HH, Rodriguez R, Romrell J, Pitts T, Wheeler-Hegland KM, Sapienza CM. Aspiration and swallowing in Parkinson disease and rehabilitation with EMST: a randomized trial. Neurology. 2010;75(21):1912–9. https://doi.org/10.1212/WNL.0b013e3181fef115.

Tutuian R, Elton JP, Castell DO, Gideon RM, Castell JA, Katz PO. Effects of position on oesophageal function: studies using combined manometry and multichannel intraluminal impedance. Neurogastroenterol Motil. 2003;15(1):63–7. https://doi.org/10.1046/j.1365-2982.2003.00387.x.

van der Molen L, van Rossum MA, Burkhead LM, Smeele LE, Rasch CR, Hilgers FJ. A randomized preventive rehabilitation trial in advanced head and neck cancer patients treated with chemoradiotherapy: feasibility, compliance, and short-term effects. Dysphagia. 2011;26(2):155–70. https://doi.org/10.1007/s00455-010-9288-y.

Vasant DH, Michou E, O'Leary N, Vail A, Mistry S, Hamdy S. Greater Manchester stroke research network. Pharyngeal electrical stimulation in dysphagia poststroke: a prospective, randomized single-blinded interventional study. Neurorehabil Neural Repair. 2016;30(9):866–75. https://doi.org/10.1177/1545968316639129.

Welch MV, Logemann JA, Rademaker AW, Kahrilas PJ. Changes in pharyngeal dimensions effected by chin tuck. Arch Phys Med Rehabil. 1993;74(2):178–81.

Whelan K. Inadequate fluid intakes in dysphagic acute stroke. Clin Nutr. 2001;20(5):423–8. https://doi.org/10.1054/clnu.2001.0467.

White KT, Easterling C, Roberts N, Wertsch J, Shaker R. Fatigue analysis before and after shaker exercise: physiologic tool for exercise design. Dysphagia. 2008;23(4):385–91. https://doi.org/10.1007/s00455-008-9155-2.

Yoon WL, Khoo JK, Rickard Liow SJ. Chin tuck against resistance (CTAR): new method for enhancing suprahyoid muscle activity using a Shaker-type exercise. Dysphagia. 2014;29(2):243–8. https://doi.org/10.1007/s00455-013-9502-9.

The Meal of the Person with Dysphagia 5

Meals occupy an important time in the daily life of people, and as observed, they have a number of meanings that continue to retain their value when swallowing is difficult. For a dysphagic patient, eating is not less important than for a person without swallowing difficulties, and this is also true for subjects who are non-orally fed (Box 5.1). In these cases, even if there is no nutritional need, the patient wants to eat, not out of hunger but for the pleasure of eating. This desire is even increased in patients subjected to dietary restrictions to the point that, sometimes, they engage in extremely dangerous behaviors such as eating in secret, usually hastily and in unusual postures. Here we analyze the conditions required to ensure the safety of the meal of dysphagic patients and explore the possibility of palliative feeding, that is, a type of feeding devoid of nutritional meaning, with the sole purpose of satisfying the non-nutritional aspects of food. Too often dysphagic patients report consuming their meals in solitude, due to the discomfort or shame of having to cough or spit during swallowing or having to assume "strange" positions.

This is an aspect to be taken into consideration so that the rehabilitation of dysphagia patients not only improves the biomechanical aspects of swallowing but also affects the restoration of daily behaviors, which positively influences the quality of life of dysphagic patients.

5.1 Quality of Life and Nutrition

The projection toward a good quality life, understood as a state of well-being, happiness, and satisfaction, has accompanied human beings most likely since their birth. The debate on quality of life has ancient roots: Aristotle.

This chapter was written by Antonio Amitrano in collaboration with speech-language therapists Marianna Antonelli, Nicoletta Bonisoli, and Chiara Bonazzi.

A. Amitrano, *Dysphagia and Nutrition*,
https://doi.org/10.1007/978-3-031-77449-2_5

Box 5.1 Non-oral Feeding Methods

Enteral nutrition (*EN*): artificial nutrition practiced through tubes positioned at the gastric or jejunal level with which a nutritional mixture is directly administered in the patient's digestive tract. EN is indicated for subjects whose gastrointestinal function is normal. The mixtures can be administered in a bolus, intermittent, continuous manner.

Parenteral nutrition (*PN*): artificial nutrition that consists of the administration via IV, central or peripheral, of nutritional substrates in a sterile form. The food substrates, not passing through the gastrointestinal channel, must necessarily be in an elementary state because they cannot be "digested," that is, subjected to the complex enzymatic-enteric system.

He dealt with it in *Nicomachean Ethics* with the concept of *eudaimonia*, "good spirit" or "happiness" in ancient Greek. Even Plato dedicated his thought and several years of his life to organizing the perfect government and city. The two Greek philosophers were then followed over the centuries by numerous other philosophers, sociologists, and religious, who have defined the constituent elements of the happy community. Today, quality of life is the result of political, social, economic, and geographical factors, bringing together a long list of indicators used by national and international agencies to study various aspects related to quality of life to compile a world ranking of countries on the basis of the quality of life of the inhabitants. The concept of "quality of life" is, at least intuitively, quite simple because the term has entered the common lexicon in many areas of daily life, and the same phrase, used especially in the English version of *quality of life* (QOL), began to be used in its modern sense from the 1960s of the twentieth century, when people began to talk about welfare, whose fundamental principles are outlined in the section on social rights of the Universal Declaration of Human Rights. Since the 1960s, QOL, mainly in the United States, has been introduced to describe the progress of society; it is no longer measured exclusively in quantitative terms, for example, according to the level of economic wealth achieved, but rather includes other indicators related to different aspects of living. From this perspective, specific measurement tools have been developed, which indicate the level of well-being achieved in a given sociocultural context (social indicators) and describe, quantifying it, the degree of well-being achieved by a population (Rapley 2003). In the last 30 years, in medical vocabulary, the use of the expression "quality of life" to define a series of aspects that go beyond strictly clinical areas has become increasingly common. In the medical context, it may not be as easy to frame the concept of quality of life, so a reflection is necessary on its roots and on the sectors of medicine where its use is most relevant. The process through which we have started to discuss quality of life in the medical field can be dated back to 1948. In that year, the World Health Organization officially defined in its statute the concept of health: a state characterized by complete physical, mental, and social well-being and not simply by the absence of disease or infirmity. This definition led to a great revolution, as it defined health as a state of well-being of the individual, broader than the correct biological functioning. In fact, disease not only damages purely biological and functional aspects of the organism but also, often, with different nuances depending on the disease itself, the personality of the subject, and the social context of reference, significantly affects the social, emotional, family-relational, and work life of the individual. Disease also changes the way the subject interprets life itself and identifies existential priorities. The concept of quality of life in the health field has therefore developed during the second half of the twentieth century in a context of profound change in Western societies, in which there has been overall growth in the average age of the population, with a consequent increase both in the prevalence of age-related diseases and in the incidence of chronic-degenerative diseases. This has put a significant part of the population in the perspective of having to live with disease, without a realistic hope of complete recovery and with the need therefore to live with the outcomes through a process of readjustment of their own reality. These elements have made it indispensable to reconceptualize the effectiveness of medical intervention. The theoretical framework of reference for medicine for many years has been a biomedical model in which every disease can be treated and health is seen as the absence of disease. Over time, such a guiding framework has become increasingly inadequate for evaluating the effectiveness of treatments and, in general, addressing the problems of modern medicine (Portney and Watkins 2007). The "objective" criterion, in short, is no longer able to respond on its own to the more complex and articulated questions posed by the new medical science.

The WHO definition of 1948, which defines health as "a state of complete physical, mental, psychological, emotional and social well-being," introduced into clinical evaluation the consideration of the subjective aspect, broadening the horizon, until then restricted, to medical aspects to the overall evaluation of quality of life. From this perspective, the patient's point of view and his or her choices in relation to the disease and its possible treatments constitute a very important aspect of the evaluation (Hartzband and Groopman 2009). According to the biopsychosocial model, health is a dynamic combination of biological and behavioral aspects, determined by many factors: health is therefore the consequence of personal and social decisions over which the individual can potentially exercise considerable control (Zucconi and Howell 2003).

Does quality of life, a fundamental concept in the description of an individual's life and health, also depend on diet? Demonstrating the relationship between quality of life and diet, in this context, will be immediately useful for including the latter category among those determining the quality of life and, later on, to support the safeguarding of diet even in extreme conditions to maintain an acceptable QOL of the subject.

When we talk about diet, we refer to two different terms: "diet" and "nutrition." First, we refer both to the act of eating, that is, to the intake of food as a vital physiological activity in response to psychic and physical hunger stimuli, and to the set of foods, which as a whole constitute the dietary regime adopted by humans. With "nutrition," on the other hand, we refer to the set of biological processes that allow humans to absorb and use all the food substances ingested, which are necessary for the survival of the organism. This aspect is closely linked to health and therefore to quality of life; in fact, the relationships among nutrition, health, and quality of life have been known since ancient times. The importance and close link of the pair "diet and good health" are underlined by the World Health Organization (WHO), which considers adequate nutrition and health to be fundamental rights. Diet is one of the factors that most affects the development, performance, and productivity of people; the quality of life; and the psycho-physical conditions with which aging is faced (INRAN 2003). The analysis of the paths and processes related to food has highlighted, toward the end of the twentieth century, the importance of some diets for leading a healthy life and preventing diseases and infirmities. In this context, the centrality of the so-called Mediterranean diet, now a heritage of humanity protected by UNESCO, was affirmed.

In 1945, a contingent of Americans landed at Salerno, among whom was the scientist Ancel Keys. During his stay in Italy, he noticed that the inhabitants of the area had an almost total absence of cardiovascular diseases, compared with the population of his country of origin. Keys hypothesized that the secret lies in the quality of the food consumed: this healthy lifestyle, or this way of eating, was precisely defined as "Mediterranean diet," and Keys studied the different eating habits in Italy and the United States to demonstrate the clear correlation between diet and the incidence of certain diseases. The Mediterranean diet began to be considered an ideal food model for health. To further verify this hypothesis, various studies have been conducted, the most famous of which is the *Seven Countries Study*, which compared the eating habits, lifestyle, and incidence of certain diseases in seven countries: from 1958 to 1970, the eating habits, lifestyle, and health status, indicated by various clinical parameters, of a sample of over 12,000 men aged between 40 and 59 years from Italy, Yugoslavia, Greece, the Netherlands, Finland, the United States, and Japan were monitored. The results of this important study constitute the first real step in relating the incidence of cardiovascular diseases to the consumption of different types of fats (saturated, monounsaturated, and polyunsaturated), cholesterol levels, and lifestyles. The outcome of this study highlighted, among other aspects, that the eating habits observed in Italy and Greece (especially in coastal areas) were the healthiest among all those examined.

All over the world, the Mediterranean diet is always synonymous with healthy eating because it is capable of keeping the body healthy, preventing many diseases, and providing long-term expectations of healthy life. In 2010, it was recognized by UNESCO as "intangible cultural heritage of humanity" and was rated as the best, precisely owing to the daily presence of generous portions of spaghetti, bread, oil, wine, legumes, etc. Nutrition is therefore almost exclusively connoted in terms of health and is closely related to quality of life.

Nutrition, which is an activity that includes the intake of food and that we can roughly coincide with the meal, pertains to the emotional relational sphere and to that of pleasure (Fischler 1990). As observed, eating, especially at mealtime, is an expression of sociability and taking part in the group. Nutrition, in its most exquisitely gastronomic sense, represents an increasingly important and significant dimension of social life and, in turn, influences other aspects of the cultural and economic context. Food is certainly one of the main sources of pleasure and well-being in contemporary societies, in many of which the problems of hunger and malnutrition have been overcome. Food is one of the most widespread and immediate sources of gratification and multisensory enjoyment. Food is savored with taste; it wraps us with its aromas, *food design*, and colors delight; and it provides the sensation of palpable materiality.

The enjoyment of food concerns various dimensions:

- *Physical*, that is, the pleasure of good eating and good drinking.
- *Cultural*, since through a gastronomical experience, you come into contact with a new culture.
- *Relational-interpersonal*, considering that the social function of food has a value comparable to the quality of what is drunk and eaten; at the table, you meet new people and reproduce defined social roles. In fact, the possibility of eating certain foods and choosing certain sites has always been a factor in distinguishing social class and has become the expression of a specific lifestyle and taste.

Food is increasingly common as a special experience, which can lead to emotion and amazement when dishes that are considered true masterworks, which are made by creative and brilliant chefs, are tasted. Of course, experiencing these sensations requires particular knowledge, as well as a certain economic capacity that allows one to attend fine restaurants. However, food can also arouse pleasure even in those who are not provided with specific preparation but can guess and perceive with their own sensitivity the value and quality of a dish. The analysis of the different areas involved in nutrition can only lead us to fully include this aspect among those on which quality of life is based, and this is relevant at all ages of life, including old age, when the value of food is even greater not only than that of a resource necessary for physical needs but also that of an element that affects the quality of individual and collective life. Foods are associated not only with health conditions but also with social participation and identity processes (Corvo and Fassino 2015). Food does not cease to have this meaning in non-self-sufficient subjects when we need to experience that others see us and appreciate us as unique individuals and not just as elements of a crowd (Aremyr 1993).

5.2 The Meal Setting

Eating is a fundamental element in determining quality of life. It is therefore essential to ensure that dysphagic subjects, who, albeit with limitations, can eat per os, have a safe and satisfying meal. Additionally, as we will see in PAR. 5.3, it is important, if desired, to guarantee the patient in terminal conditions or unable to feed per os a portion of nutrition, which no longer aims to meet nutritional needs but only to satisfy, as far as possible, the share of pleasure and sociability that feeding provides.

Patients who, at the end of the evaluation, are suitable for various levels of oral feeding, that is, with a score on the *Functional Oral Intake Scale* (FOIS) from 2 to

6, must pay attention to a series of elements during the meal to increase the level of safety:

- Posture
- The characteristics of the food
- The characteristics of the setting and the behavior of the caregiver
- Emergency management
- Oral hygiene

5.2.1 Posture

The posture assumed during a meal plays an important role in determining the degree of safety. Importantly, posture is also important in non-oral feeding; in fact during enteral feeding through a tube, patients must be seated with the trunk, forming an angle of 30–45° with the pelvis (Fig. 5.1).

This precaution is important for preventing gastric reflux which, in the case of aspiration, can cause pulmonary inflammation or *aspiration pneumonitis* (Box 5.2; Marik 2001; Son et al. 2017).

The correct posture to assume during mealtime includes the position of the head, the trunk, and, in general, the whole body. The possible alternatives to be considered are having the meal seated on a chair or in a wheelchair or even in bed. In these three different situations, specific precautions must be taken: it is important to ensure that the patient assumes the correct position and maintains it throughout mealtime. In fact, in some situations, such as when a person has meals in bed, it is possible that the proper posture is not maintained for the entire duration of the meal, thus exposing the subject to greater risks, especially toward the end of the meal, which is generally the most delicate moment, due to the onset of fatigue or distraction.

Box 5.2 Aspiration Pneumonia

The passage of food material into the lower airways can lead to the onset of aspiration pneumonia. The aspirated material can come from the mouth or from the stomach. The term *aspiration pneumonia* refers to the aspiration of secretions or infected food from the mouth and upper airways, whereas aspiration *pneumonitis* is caused by the aspiration of sterile material of gastric origin (Marik 2001; Son et al. 2017).

When a patient with dysphagia consumes his meal while sitting on a chair, he should sit upright, with comfortable forearm support and feet firmly on the ground. The center of gravity of the pelvis should be equally balanced over both buttocks and the hip flexed at 90°. A tubular foam cushion or a rolled towel placed under the knees can prevent the pelvis from sliding forward and helps to maintain a correct posture throughout the meal. The head is in a central position, with the gaze facing

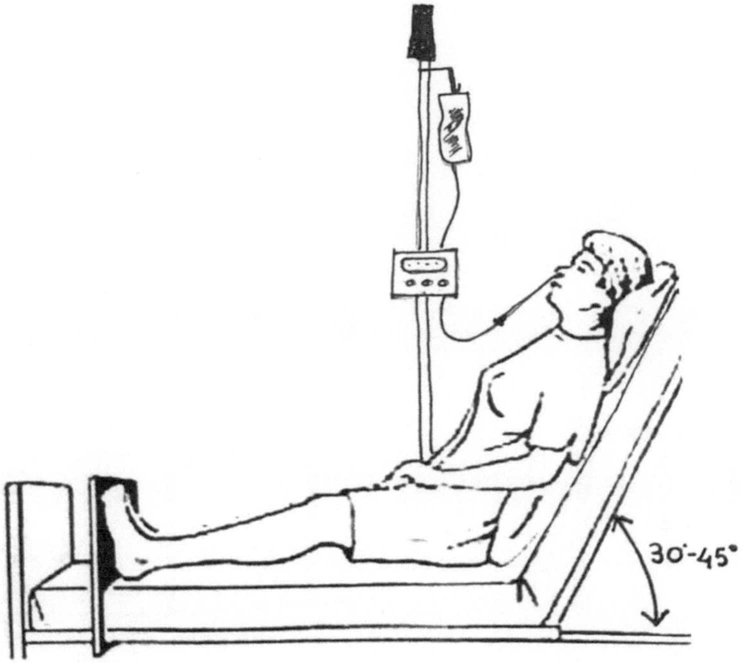

Fig. 5.1 Correct position for enteral nutrition. (Drawing by Cecilia Amitrano)

forward: this position is considered neutral for the adoption of postures indicated from time to time by the speech therapist as compensation to adapt during the meal. The arms rest on the thighs; in the case of instability of the trunk, it is advisable to rest the forearms on a table in front of the patient. The height of the chair should be adequate to allow the feet to be well supported on the ground and consequently to bend the joints of the knees and hips at 90° (Fig. 5.2).

Even the patient who eats while sitting in a wheelchair must observe the described position. Of particular importance is the stabilization of the trunk, facilitated by the backrest of the wheelchair itself, which must have a proper inclination, possibly to be corrected with cushions. The arms help in assuming the right position by the armrests and the worktable, which can be applied to the front of the wheelchair (Fig. 5.3). If the subject does not independently control the posture of the head, headrests can be used, which are chosen in the appropriate shape, even with the help of buckles or elastic straps, to maintain the correct position of the head for the entire duration of the meal. It is also important to observe the position of the footrests, which must ensure the possibility of good foot support and consequently flexion at 90° of the knees. Finally, the correct position of the legs significantly affects the position of the entire body.

The position in bed, which is where the majority of patients in acute hospitals consume their meals, is particularly delicate. The backrest of the bed should be raised to 90° to bring the hip as much as possible to bend at a right angle. The legs

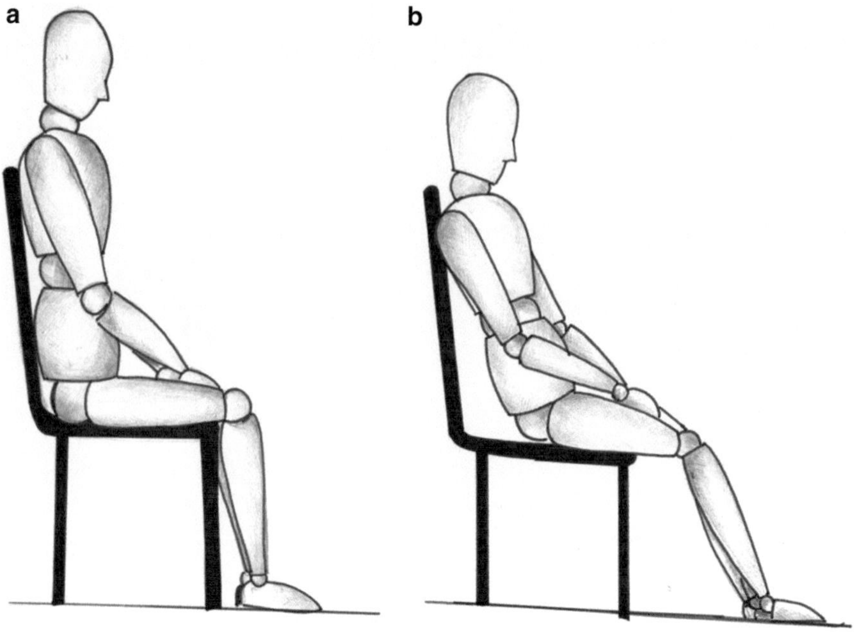

Fig. 5.2 Position during meals: (**a**) correct sitting; (**b**) incorrect sitting. (Drawing by Cecilia Amitrano)

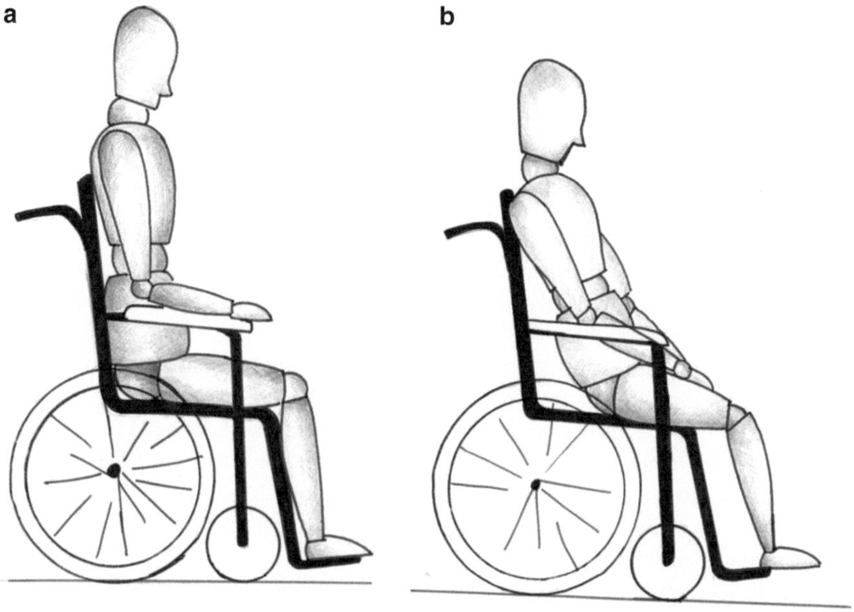

Fig. 5.3 Position during meals for the patient in a wheelchair: (**a**) correct sitting; (**b**) incorrect sitting. (Drawing by Cecilia Amitrano)

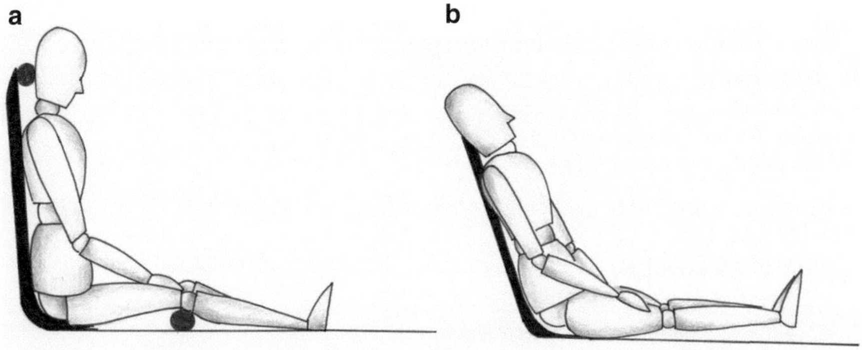

Fig. 5.4 Position during meals consumed in bed: (**a**) correct sitting; (**b**) incorrect sitting. (Drawing by Cecilia Amitrano)

are stretched on the bed, with a roll or a cushion placed under the knees, and raised by approximately 30° to avoid the pelvis from sliding forward during a meal (Fig. 5.4). A front table facilitates the support of the forearms. In the case of nonreclining beds, which are not recommended for use with dysphagic patients, it is possible to achieve the sitting position by adding overlapping layers of cushions between the bed's headboard and the patient's back. It is also useful to place a small pillow or a rolled towel behind the neck to support the cervical section of the spine and thus avoid dangerous extensions of the head.

5.2.2 The Characteristics of Food

The choice of food for the meal of dysphagic patients involves several professionals. The nutritional aspects, which concern the determination of the specific caloric needs of the subject and the choice of nutrients that make up the diet, are the responsibility of the nutritionist and the dietician. The phoniatrist and the speech-language therapist have the task of identifying the consistency in which various nutrients should be administered. Once these choices are made, it is essential that the food arriving on the dysphagic patient's table exactly respects the given instructions. For this reason, it is important that any facility where patients eat should consider specific diets for dysphagic patients in their corporate diet. Importantly the kitchen team who prepares the meals must be adequately informed about the specific characteristics of diets for dysphagia and the importance of paying attention to homogeneity and the adherence of the prepared foods to the speech therapist's indications. Taking into account textures, the patient's preferences must be considered, and particular care must be given as far as the variability of the foods is concerned. One of the main problems of modified consistency diets is acceptance by patients: several studies highlight that modified consistency diets are among the main causes of malnutrition in institutionalized elderly people (Box 5.3; Vucea et al. 2018; Scalmani et al. 2000).

Box 5.3 Elements that Contribute to Malnutrition in Institutionalized Elderly Individuals

- Diet changes
- Decrease in privacy (rituals, choices, *mealtime*)
- Decrease in caloric *intake*
- Medical diagnosis (dementia, stroke, etc.)
- Mental state
- Medication intake
- Physical impediments
- Sensory changes related to age (decrease in taste)

These findings suggest the use of modified consistency diets exclusively in situations where they are indispensable for ensuring meal safety. In other cases, resorting to practicable alternatives, respecting safety and nutritional efficacy criteria, is useful. For example, in edentulous subjects, for whom a solid consistency diet should be avoided, this does not necessarily have to be replaced by a creamy diet, but a minced diet can be used, in which the individual pieces do not exceed the safety dimensions indicated by the IDDSI. In a hypothetical ground diet, meatballs do not fall within this category, which, although composed of ground elements, are considered solid because of the cohesion of the individual elements. On the other hand, a ragout, in which the chopped meat keeps its constituent elements, could wholly fall into a ground diet. Particular care must then be dedicated to the palatability of the foods included in the modified consistency diets. The term "palatable" defines a food that is "good to the palate," tasty, and of pleasant consistency and that gives particular satisfaction in eating it. Palatable foods can be the fattest because aromatic molecules are liposoluble; therefore, they are better conveyed to the mouth by a fatty matrix. This characteristic, which is well known and widely used by the food industry engaged in producing *comfort food*, can be the key, if properly managed under the supervision of a nutritionist, to increase the acceptability of modified consistency diets (Box 5.4).

Box 5.4 Comfort Food

Comfort food refers to any food provided with a consoling, nostalgic, and/or sentimental value. *Comfort food* cuddles us: whether it is made up of genuine food or junk food, it reminds us of childhood and warms our hearts in our life's bad moments.

In the administration of foods, especially those with a creamy consistency, the color and flavor characteristics of individual foods must be maintained. For this reason, mixing several foods together should be avoided, thus creating dishes with color and flavor that are not very appealing.

5.2.2.1 Food and 3D Printers: The New Frontier for Food

The first 3D printer, a machine that reproduces a virtual model in the real world, was created by a researcher at Columbia University, Jonathan Blutinger. Common 3D printers use plastic materials that, once melted, are expelled through nozzles that produce overlapping layers of material, which, once solidified, constitute the final object. Recently, 3D printing devices have entered the market that can also be used to "print" food. The operating principle of the 3D printer for food continues to be based on the laser, which, in this case, is used not to print objects but food. The plastic or other materials, which are usually used in this type of sprinter, are replaced by the ingredients necessary to make the desired dish. Food 3D printers work with the same method, but instead of treating plastic materials in coils, they use food, which is generally reduced to dough. Owing to the laser, the food produced by the printer is hot and needs a short passage in the oven before being consumed. To make a dish with the 3D printer, it is necessary to reduce the ingredients to dough and insert them into the appropriate containers, from where they come out through nozzles designed for this purpose, creating, by overlapping layers, the desired dish. The foods that are most suitable for treatment with this technology are sauces and creams, which turn into dishes very quickly, and owing to their high definition, they present very well. Owing to the ease of preparation with 3D technology, foods adapt surprisingly to individual tastes and allow a high degree of variability. The appropriate containers of the printer can contain raw or cooked ingredients, which do not undergo any alterations in taste or nutritional properties during the printing process. 3D printers create food of shapes that can also completely deviate from the original ones: think about the possibility, especially in children's nutrition, of giving original shapes to foods that are generally not liked, which in this way increases their appeal. Among the advantages of using a 3D printer in the kitchen is therefore the possibility of personalizing meals, not only in shape but also in the content of different nutrients, such as vitamins and even calories, starting from a base dough formulated on the needs of the person who will eat it. 3D technology is very promising for the packaging of food for dysphagic subjects. In fact, starting from creamy doughs, you can create dishes that, in taste and aesthetics, do not differ from the corresponding solids (Figs. 5.5 and 5.6).

5.2.3 The Characteristics of the Setting and the Behavior of the Caregiver

The setting in which dysphagic patients have meals must be quiet and free from sources of distraction: turning off television and any other device, which can cause distraction, is recommended. In particular, it is necessary to turn off the TV when it is in an overhead position on suspended arms, as is common in hospital rooms. In these cases, the patient would risk eating with his head extended, a posture that, as we have observed, if on the one hand, improves the progression of the bolus in the oral cavity and, on the other hand, increases the risk of aspiration. The environment in which one eats needs to be quiet, and it is important for the

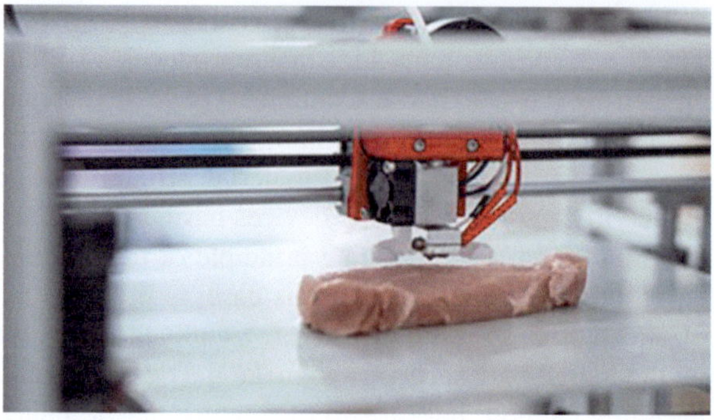

Fig. 5.5 Steak made with a 3D printer

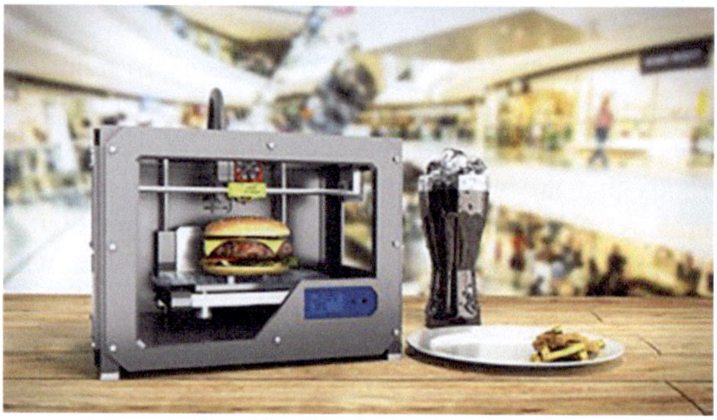

Fig. 5.6 Sandwich made with a 3D printer

caregiver to limit their verbal interventions to the time space between bites, avoiding questions such as: "Is it good?" "Do you like it?" "Is it hot?" Asking a question is a strong stimulation to speak: the two functions, the articulatory and the swallowing functions, employ the same anatomical structures, which, however, must be used at different times to avoid dangerous overlaps. "When you eat you do not talk and when you talk you do not eat" is a saying enclosing a fundamental safety criterion of feeding. To feed dysphagic patients, the use of special cutlery made of suitable materials that are fit for the difficulties of gripping may be effective. In these cases, one can create personalized grips in thermoplastic materials. Special plates and glasses are also available. If patients have bite reflex, plastic cutlery that can break and metal cutlery that can injure the patient should be avoided. In these cases, the use of rubber or thick plastic cutlery, which does not yield pressure on the bite, is recommended. In the case of dysphagia caused by liquids, flute beak glasses and containers with a longer edge or a groove that allows one to drink even with the head in forward flexion are helpful.

A useful alternative to flute beak glasses can be cups or wide diameter glasses, which equally allow emptying without extending the head; however, long and narrow glasses are avoided (Fig. 5.7). Whenever the sole forward flexed head posture is not sufficient to reduce difficulties in taking liquids, thickeners can be used, i.e., starches or gums, which, when added to water, change their consistency. Importantly drinking from a straw is not facilitating because it implements a more complex

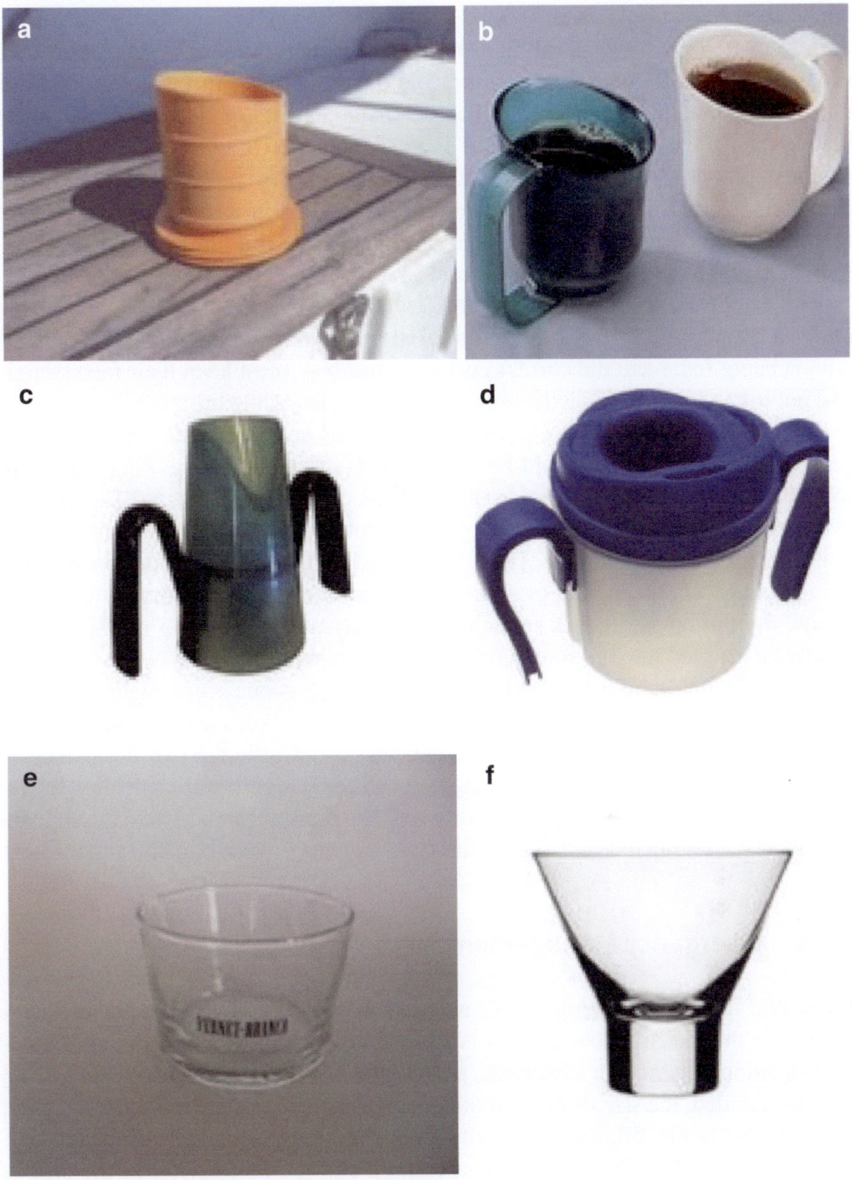

Fig. 5.7 Models of glasses suitable for hydrating patients with dysphagia

motor scheme than does drinking from a glass. Each time, it will therefore be necessary to evaluate whether the use of a straw can actually be helpful for the patient. It is also useful to remember that drinking with a straw makes it difficult to control the volume of the bolus, a strategy that, in some patients, solves the problems of swallowing liquids. A separate discussion is required for the use of a syringe: generally, when the squirt is used, which is filled with liquid or semiliquid, but more difficultly with semisolid, it can be a valid aid in feeding certain dysphagic patients, if used correctly. It is absolutely necessary to avoid the use of the squirt to insert food into the patient's mouth, except to introduce small amounts of liquid or semiliquid under the tongue, in the part anterior to the lingual frenulum. In other words, the squirt should approach the lips not in a horizontal but in a vertical position so that from top to bottom, small volume of bolus should be deposited in the anterior floor of the mouth. If used correctly, therefore, the squirt is very useful for controlling the volume of the bolus introduced into the oral cavity.

The caregiver or the health personnel who feed patients unable to feed themselves are considered part of the setting (Bonazzi and Amitrano 2012). The patient who is being fed, once the correct posture is reached, must keep their face straight and not rotate it to approach the cutlery. The assistant, while bringing the cutlery to the patient's mouth, must be careful not to lead his head in a backward movement of extension. The spoon should be inserted into the mouth in the direction of the long diameter and then removed in the direction of the short diameter. This helps to avoid extension of the head, which generally occurs to prevent the handle of the cutlery from touching the nose. The bolus should be placed, in the indicated amount, in the front part of the mouth, preferably under the tongue. It is important to observe a slow rhythm or one that is suitable for the patient's swallowing rhythm. A bite should be inserted into the mouth only when the previous bite has been swallowed. Additionally, one should not drink during a meal unless one is completely sure that the mouth is empty. In fact, the introduction of a liquid bolus into the oral cavity in the presence of boluses of other consistencies would generate two consistencies, which, as has been previously reported, constitute a significant criticality for the successful completion of the swallowing act. The assistant should not stimulate the person who is eating to speak or ask questions except between one bite and the next.

5.2.4 Emergency Management

It is useful for those assisting people with dysphagia to understand the behaviors to observe in the case of choking. This is a possible eventuality, although not frequent if prevention criteria are observed: small bites should be provided and stringy cheeses avoided, the size of the individual parts of the food should not exceed those indicated by the IDDSI, the rhythm of feeding and eating should be slow, and multiple bites should not be allowed to accumulate in the oral cavity. In the case of choking, it is advisable not to panic so as not to worsen the understandable state of agitation of the person who is choking. In such moments, it is not useful to make the person who is choking drink, nor to pat them on the back or make them raise their arms. First, the mouth should be opened to check for the presence of food residues or a dental prosthesis, which, if dislodged, could obstruct the oral cavity. Only if the residues are easily reachable from the outside should one proceed with their removal; when, instead, they are well lodged in the throat, it is better not to attempt their removal to avoid pushing them further in. If the subject is standing and still conscious, the Heimlich maneuver should be performed, named after the American doctor Henry Heimlich, who first described it in 1974. The maneuver can also be performed by nonmedical personnel, but it is always advisable, in the event of choking episodes, to immediately alert emergency services by calling 118. Once positioned behind the patient, the rescuer uses their hands and arms to exert a series of rapid and deep pressures on the abdominal area, specifically between the sternum and the navel. The thrust is directed upward to compress the diaphragm, which in turn compresses the lungs which, with the expulsion of air, exert a pneumatic thrust on the obstructing body; in other words, the maneuver simulates a powerful and artificial cough. In cases where the subject is sitting on a chair or in a wheelchair, the Heimlich maneuver is performed in the same way from behind the subject. If instead the patient is unconscious, emergency services must be called extremely quickly, and in the meantime, they should be laid on their back with their head turned to the side, cleaning the mouth of any residue. Positioning oneself above the patient at the level of the thighs with one leg on each side, one proceeds to place the hands crossed between the navel and the sternum and to exert rapid and decisive compressions until the resumption of breathing. In the case of obese subjects or pregnant women, the procedure remains the same, except for the compressions, which, in these cases, should be performed by pressing energetically on the lower middle third of the sternum, approximately 5 cm above the xiphoid process. It is necessary to train in the execution of the maneuver with the many tutorials available online by the Italian Red Cross (CRI) and the *European Resuscitation Council* (ERC) or even better by attending appropriate training courses at accredited institutions. The new ERC guidelines provide for alternating five subdiaphragmatic compressions and five back blows between the shoulder blades. These are performed with the open palm of the hand between the two shoulder blades with a lateral escape route. The patient's torso is flexed forward with the bending line possibly at the level of the hips. In this way, the rescuer uses both arms: one arm is positioned transversely at the level of the hips and serves as a bending axis for the patient, whereas the other applies firm blows with a lateral escape route between the shoulder blades. The measures described are to be implemented in the case of choking in adult subjects; the maneuvers to be used in the case of choking in infants and children are different and specific. Given the life-saving value of these maneuvers, it is useful for anyone assisting a dysphagic patient to practice their execution by attending specific courses and, in any case, to ask their doctor for clarification on anything unclear in our description.

5.2.5 Oral Hygiene

Oral hygiene is the cleaning of the oral cavity and in a broader sense the set of maneuvers necessary to maintain it. Proper oral hygiene positively affects quality of life. A healthy mouth promotes not only chewing but also sociability, affecting speech and smile, which are important elements of social life. Research consistently indicates that oral health has a significant effect on quality of life (Almomani et al. 2006; Chalmers et al. 2002; Petersen et al. 2005; Sheiham 2005; Watt 2005). Conversely, poor oral hygiene is correlated with halitosis; bleeding gums; tooth damage and loss; worsening physical appearance, self-esteem, and social relationships; worsening swallowing and articulation; a reduction in food intake; weight loss; discomfort; pain; and overall behavioral change (Australian Government Department of Social Services 2009). Furthermore, in dysphagic patients, the aspiration of infectious agents in the oropharyngeal tract remains the most common route of infection of the lower respiratory tract (Scannapieco et al. 2003). Some authors indicate poor oral hygiene as one of the major causes of aspiration pneumonia in nursing homes (Quagliarello et al. 2005): out of the 613 patients assisted in nursing homes, among the 9 parameters investigated (poor oral hygiene, difficulty swallowing, lack of influenza vaccination, depression, active smoking, food intake posture, intake of sedatives, antacids, angiotensin converting enzyme), poor oral hygiene and difficulty swallowing are the only elements that are significantly correlated with the onset of aspiration pneumonia. It has been estimated that in a hospital, the cost for the prevention of nosocomial pneumonia is less than 10% of the cost associated with the treatment of a single case (Lux 2006). One study identified dental plaque as the site of pathogens of the lower respiratory tract (Sumi et al. 2007). Regular oral hygiene can prevent the onset of aspiration pneumonia (Bartlett et al. 1974). The knowledge acquired on the relationship between oral hygiene and aspiration pneumonia has not led to a substantial improvement in the care of institutionalized patients receiving oral hygiene. An American study, which was carried out on a population of institutionalized elderly individuals and replicated approximately 20 years apart, highlighted a lack of oral hygiene in both cases (Weyant et al. 1993; Bassim et al. 2008). In a systematic review, it was estimated that approximately one in ten deaths from aspiration pneumonia could be avoided with better oral hygiene (Sjögren et al. 2008).

The evaluation of the mouth precedes the provision of oral care: the use of direct light allows the oral cavity to be evaluated, leaving room for better visualization. There are also numerous tooth brushing techniques, although there are no clear indications of the superiority of one method over another (Asadoorian and Locker 2006). It is important to brush the teeth systematically and completely, via an appropriate technique.

Dentures need suitable care, as they are potential reservoirs of plaque and pathogenic bacteria (Sumi et al. 2002). Oral hygiene requires various tools (Fig. 5.8), such as the following:

- Hands and individual fingers
- Tongue depressors, oral sponges, toothbrushes, finger toothbrushes, toothbrushes applicable to the suction probe, tongue cleaners, and specific wipes soaked for oral hygiene
- Liquid oral lubricants, sprays, gels (also butter, olive oil, paraffin oil, Vaseline, and lip balm), aromatic substances, ice, mouthwashes, antibacterial emollients/moisturizers, and artificial saliva
- Toothpastes with/without foam

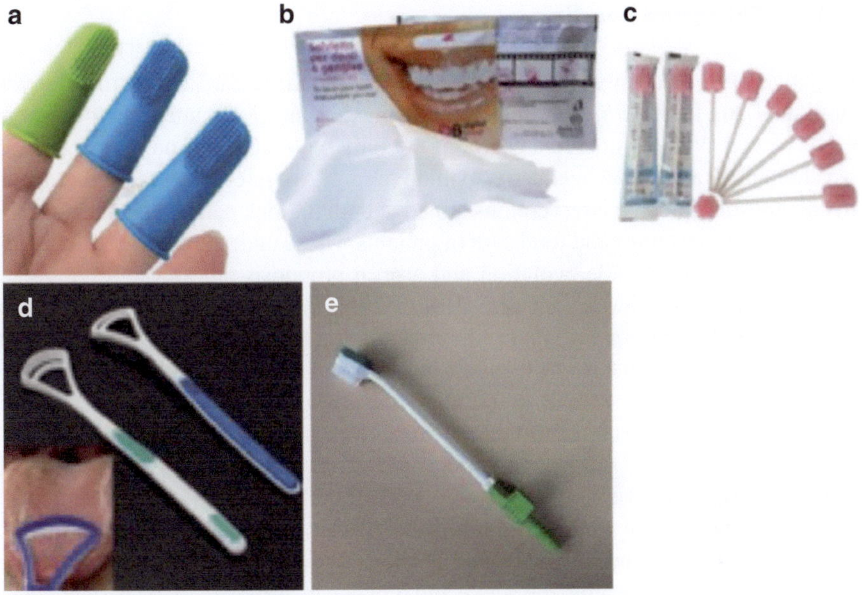

Fig. 5.8 Tools for oral hygiene. (**a**) Finger toothbrush; (**b**) moistened wipes for oral hygiene; (**c**) sponge swabs; (**d**) tongue cleaner; (**e**) toothbrush applicable to a suction system

Cleaning should be carried out several times a day to keep the mouth clean and healthy. Oral hygiene is particularly recommended for certain types of patients. Patients on artificial nutrition (EN and TPN), not using the mouth for feeding, are at greater risk of deterioration of oral conditions. It should also be considered that in patients who have oral breathing, this contributes to the drying out of the mucous membranes, with the consequent hardening of any secretions present in the mouth. In addition, the presence of oxygen therapy contributes to the drying of mucous membranes, making their systematic lubrication of primary importance.

The procedure requires the following:

- Always explain to the patient what is being done.
- Position the patient in bed, sitting at least 40°, with the head and shoulders supported.
- Use clear and non-hesitant touch (different modes might communicate insecurity and discomfort).
- Start from the cheeks, chin, and lip contour, and proceed progressively toward the inside of the mouth, as far as possible.
- Utmost attention should be given to the presence of the bite reflex. In the execution of oral hygiene procedures, the operator must preserve their own health by wearing the necessary personal protection devices (PPE).

5.3 Palliative Feeding

Palliative feeding falls within the broader field of palliative care, a term that derives from the Latin term *pallium* ("cloak"), and indicates the global attention to the person. The patient is considered a bearer of not only physical needs but also spiritual, psychological, and social needs. By "palliative care," we refer to the set of therapeutic, diagnostic, and care interventions aimed at both the sick person and their family unit, aimed at the active and total care of patients whose underlying disease, characterized by an unstoppable evolution and a grim prognosis, no longer responds to specific treatments (law 15 March 2010, n. 38, art. 2). Palliative care intervenes when the goal of care is no longer literal healing, as in *restitutio ad integrum*, but becomes the improvement of the quality of the remaining life, with the awareness that an irreversible process of preparation for death has been established. In the practice of palliative care, attention also extends to the family unit of the sick person, which also needs support and assistance (from the Latin *adsistere*, "to stand by") globally. Palliative care consists of professional medical, nursing, rehabilitative, and psychological services, nursing help, professional guardianship assistance, and spiritual support and is aimed not only at cancer patients but also at all incurable patients. They also constitute the active and global care provided to the patient when the disease no longer responds to therapies aimed at healing and has an interdisciplinary character, involving the patient, their family, and the community in general. Their purpose is not to accelerate or delay death but to preserve the best possible quality of life until the end, as indicated by the *European Association for Palliative Care* (EAPC). Nutrition and eating contribute to the quality of life of a person. The act of nourishing oneself consists not only of providing the caloric intake that the body needs but also of the spheres of pleasure, care, tradition, home, and family. In situations where nourishing the body with balanced hydroelectrolytic intake is no longer a "sufficient" element to best face the disease and fight it until healing, the need for nutrition transforms, bringing to the fore the other meanings that food has. At such times, food once again reveals the multiplicity of its meanings: it is much more than just the food necessary for our body for sustenance; it is an expression of friendship and love, a means of emotional and social relationships, capable of creating emotions and bringing back distant memories. Palliative nutrition is dedicated to those who are in terminal condition or in a situation of severe and irreversible dysphagia. In these cases, albeit with different meanings, nutrition is ensured enterally or parenterally, methods that exclude the use of the mouth for nutrition and somehow eliminate the communicative-relational and hedonistic meanings of food. In such situations, the loss of the ability to feed by mouth is considered real bereavement (Amitrano 2019), which concerns not only the patient but also the whole family, who is deprived of the role of care under this condition. Food and eating are important elements of emotional relationships and are expressed in various forms of care. Replacing a bag of preparation in an infusion pump is not comparable to preparing food for a relative. Nutrition represents a central element in the care of the sick person, and even in cases where nutrition is no longer strictly necessary, the concept of "care," including psychological, continues to attribute great importance to food. The food prepared by those who love us, even if it is overcooked, bland, or hard, is the best nourishment for the soul. It therefore becomes important to find the least risky way to get the patient, who expressly requests it, to consume minimal amounts of the foods they want to eat or drink. The risk of patients being exposed to such particular situations by having them consume minimal amounts of food or drinks that they have expressly requested constitutes an increase in the qualitative aspects of everyday life. The possible risks, which in any case must be minimized by adopting all possible precautions, should not deny the fulfilment of the desire of a person who is going through the last stretch of their earthly life or who will no longer be able to recover swallowing. The German National Medical Association explained in 2004 and reiterated in 2011 that "End-of-life assistance consists of applying palliative care and therefore also in supporting and providing basic assistance. It does not always include the artificial administration of liquids and food, as this could represent a heavy burden for terminally ill patients. Hunger and thirst as subjective sensations must instead be treated" (Bundesärztekammer 2004). In the terminal phase, to quell the sensation of hunger and thirst, it is more than sufficient to administer liquids and food in minimal quantities (Borasio 2015). In such contexts, the role of the speech therapist is to find the most suitable way to meet the patient's needs as safely as possible. It is not possible to indicate general intervention methods because each case requires specific solutions that, once identified, must be shared and accepted by the patient and/or his care and family.

5.3.1 Speech Therapy Assistance for Oncological Patients in Palliative Care

Neoplastic disease interferes with eating behavior (Mercadante and Ripamonti 2002). Anorexic behaviors can manifest themselves already at the time of diagnosis. The lack of food intake can manifest itself as follows:

- Altered food intake, especially in patients with head-neck or digestive tract tumors.
- Nausea and vomiting are connected to chemotherapeutic and analgesic treatment.
- Actinic alterations of the pharyngeal musculature.

During illness, various aspects related to nutrition change and can turn eating—a natural, automatic, and pleasant act—into a very difficult and unpleasant process. A lower intake of food with consequent weight loss increases the level of concern of the person and especially of the family members involved in care, despite the care and efforts dedicated to their relative, thus inducing them to experience a feeling of helplessness and mourning (Mercadante and Ripamonti 2002; Prandi 2015). Certain diseases, especially in the most advanced stages, regardless of food intake, still cause gradual weight loss and increasingly severe weakening of the body (Provinciali et al. 2016). Oral feeding, as long as possible, even for hedonistic purposes, should be maintained both for the well-being and oral-buccal functionality of the patient and to support, through the symbolic meaning of food, the bond of the affective relationship between caregiver and patient. To this end, within the team dealing with palliative care, the speech therapist can be significant, training, educating, and supporting the patient and caregiver with respect to swallowing problems (Martins and Castro 2017; O'Reilly and Walshe 2015). Rehabilitation aims to enable a person with disabilities to achieve the best quality of life on a physical, functional, social, and emotional level, within the limits of their impairment and available resources. The rehabilitative process, therefore, involves a direct focus, not only on strictly clinical aspects but also on psychological and social aspects, which also include the patient's family and loved ones. There are close interconnections between the rehabilitative approach to people with disabilities and palliative care for terminally ill patients; both of them, in fact, share the same objectives, have the same therapeutic approach, and have a multidisciplinary care model, which aims to improve comfort and patient function. However, the goal of recovering some functions in patients with severe psychophysical frailty may seem controversial. It is therefore important that the therapist, called upon to intervene with this type of patient, always has a clear understanding of the motivation for his intervention and the way in which he intends to achieve the objectives he sets for himself. Among the functions that can gradually be lost, in addition to the swallowing function, there are also communicative-linguistic functions, which can be involved, regardless of the site of the primary lesion, due to the secondary effects of tumors and their treatments. The speech therapist, a health professional who performs activities aimed at prevention, treatment, rehabilitation, and functional evaluation procedures for language, communication, and swallowing disorders, can make important contributions to the palliative patient, his family, and the team that takes care of him (Kelly et al. 2018). To date, there is still little literature supporting the engagement of speech therapists in palliative care; however, the need to do so is increasingly emerging in clinical and care contexts. Nutrition and hydration are of absolute importance in patient management, both in the early and advanced stages of the disease. Nutritional aspects, in fact, are an integral part of the so-called support therapies in palliative care or pain therapy. Hyporexia and difficulty in feeding, up to cachexia, are symptoms that often cause deep suffering to patients and their relatives, as the value of health, "well-being," and conviviality that food usually assumes is lacking. Weight loss occurs due to inadequate feeding/swallowing, and the progression of the pathological process exerts great emotional pressure on the final stage of the patient's life and his or her relatives. The disease process is irreversible and can no longer be influenced or improved with food; for this reason, it is necessary for healthcare professionals to support patients and caregivers in explanations of possible palliative feeding and/or nutrition. In particular, the speech therapist, in reference to his professional skills, will have to sensitize and inform, through counselling, the caregiver and the patient about possible remedial and compensatory strategies aimed at promoting oral feeding as long as possible or possible feeding for hedonistic use (palliative feeding, in fact). The speech therapist's care intervention also aims to monitor oral complications following the evolution of the disease and/or following radiation or chemoradiation therapy to which the patient is subjected for better patient compliance with care and a positive impact on quality of life. The perception of pain, especially chronic pain, is modified by the patient's judgment of the care they receive. The interaction between the speech therapist and the terminal patient reduces the perception of his own swallowing difficulties, improving, as much as possible, the emotional state of the subject. In this sense, the patient will feel accompanied and supported in the disease process, as he is informed about possible difficulties and complications during meal intake and possible strategies to be implemented. The speech therapist's task is to monitor the patient's swallowing function, keeping an eye on possible risks of dysphagia in the evolution of the underlying disease. The functional evaluation allows the planning of appropriate interventions that are proportional to the needs and wishes of the patient and implementation of compensatory strategies and shared dietary consistency modifications, which ensure that the person can have a safe meal from a functional and psychological point of view. The speech therapist will therefore have the technical and human skills to accompany the person and his relatives in the transition from oral feeding to enteral and/or parenteral feeding, comparable to a real and proper grieving process (Amitrano 2019). It is known that appetite decreases as the disease progresses, but by using multiple strategies, it is possible to counteract the patient's increasing lack of appetite. During the course of treatment, which may also involve pain therapies, it is important not to burden the patient with a lack of appetite or to force him to eat; rather, it is advisable to gently encourage him to eat. In the event of a lack of appetite and a rapid feeling of fullness, the following is suggested:

- Serve small and often attractive meals in a relaxed atmosphere and environment.
- Distribute high-nutrient-density snacks carefully throughout the day.
- Eat meals with other people, as seeing others eat means eating.
- Proposal of foods that stimulate appetite.
- Avoid compact dishes, such as stew, or fatty and gassy products.
- Favor liquid foods, which induce a feeling of less satiety and allow easier eating.
- Remove from sight meals and products that are not consumed immediately.

The sense of hunger varies throughout the day and, generally, is greater in the first part of the day; therefore, it is useful to take advantage of breakfast and lunch to encourage patients to consume liked foods. In addition, it is important to distribute small meals more times a day. Hydration is equally important, as it promotes the elimination of toxins and the maintenance of the skin and mucous membranes. As with food, patients should not be persistently persuaded to drink but should be encouraged only to consume liquids. Drinking is recommended away from meals to promote absorption while preventing the liquids themselves from mixing with food to create a sense of satiety. To encourage the intake of liquids, patients' tastes should be taken into account by making their favorite drinks available. Ice creams, popsicles, and nutritious drinks should be included in the diet, thus improving the intake of liquids. Even for hydration, as for food, as the disease progresses, it may be advisable to change habits, for example, drinking liquids with a straw or with modified glass, depending on the difficulty encountered. The market provides a variety of fruit or chocolate-flavored preparations with high energy content, which are specifically designed for patients suffering from debilitating diseases. They are easily available in pharmacies or can be requested by a competent doctor for patients in home care. In cancer patients, it is always necessary, before taking supplements, to obtain the doctor's opinion. The patient's sense of taste can change as the disease progresses, and consequently, the experience of taste may no longer correspond to the previous perception; therefore, it is no longer possible to provide a reliable answer to the request to indicate what is liked. In light of these premises, it may be useful to vary flavors and tastes, and the following is suggested:

- Invite the patient to chew longer, because in this way, the taste might improve.
- Avoid foods with strong smells.
- Adapt food to new taste preferences.
- Pair meat dishes with sweet and fresh sauces (e.g., apple sauce or fruit compote).
- Use cold dishes, which spread less smells than hot dishes do.
- Serve foods with a mild taste, such as potatoes, white bread, toast, crackers, porridge, spreadable cheese, biscuits, and egg-and-butter cakes.
- Use aromatic herbs, sauces, or spices such as ginger, sambal, and wasabi.
- Food smells, cleaning products, perfumes, or tobacco smells should be avoided. If the meal is consumed in the same room where it is cooked, the room should be ventilated to promote the dispersion of smells before serving.

Since insufficient fluid intake can worsen the sensation of unpleasant taste in the mouth, the following is advisable:

- Suck on peppermint, candy, or gum.
- Taking care of oral hygiene and maintaining the integrity of the oral mucosa can prevent or combat oral mucositis and candidiasis.

Especially in patients in the advanced stage of the disease, monitoring the state of the oral cavity is necessary; oral cavity complications can indeed interfere with phonatory, feeding, and respiratory function. The alteration of the oral mucosa can be determined by local factors (dental prostheses, hyposalivation, alteration of salivary composition, alteration of oral flora, poor or inadequate oral hygiene) and systemic factors (drugs, nutritional alteration with protein and electrolyte reduction, immunosuppression, diabetes); the most frequent manifestations can be hyposalivation and xerostomia, stomatitis or mucositis, and bacterial or viral infections. Speech-language therapists can provide informative counselling to the caregiver on the typical signs and symptoms of mucositis so that timely recognition can be reported to the team. There are standardized scales for the evaluation of the oral cavity (Eilers et al. 1988), including the National Cancer Institute scale and the World Health Organization scale, both of which include five evaluation grades ranging from 0 to 4: grade 0 indicates the absence of symptoms, and grade 4 indicates the need for enteral or parenteral nutritional support. An interesting oral health screening is the Bed Oral Exam (BoE), born from the modification of the Oral

Assessment Guide (OAG) (Prendergast et al. 2013). This is an internationally validated screening tool for bedside evaluation of patients' oral health. It consists of the evaluation of eight characteristics that denote oral health, to which a score from 1 to 3 is assigned. The obtainable score therefore ranges from a minimum of 8 points, which equates to excellent oral health, to a maximum of 24 points, which corresponds to severe oral dysfunction. The simplicity and speed of use make this tool versatile and allow even nonspecific operators in the dental sector to evaluate patients' oral situation, decreasing the onset of complications due to poor oral health. The elements observed with this test are as follows:

- *Swallowing*: through the observation of a swallowing act and the verification of the presence of the gastroesophageal reflex, the operator assesses whether the patient swallows normally or has pain or difficulty or if it is not possible for them to swallow.
- *Lips*: the operator observes whether the lips are smooth and pink, dry or cracked, or ulcerated or bleeding.
- *Tongue*: whether the tongue has a pink, moist appearance, with papillae present: if it is coated, with loss of papillae; if it has a shiny appearance with or without redness; if it has blisters; if it is cracked or bleeding.
- *Saliva*: saliva is observed through the use of a tongue depressor placed in the center and on the floor of the tongue. The operator must report whether the saliva is watery, thick and viscous, or absent.
- *Mucous membranes*: whether the mucous membranes have a pink and moist appearance, if they are reddened or coated without ulceration, or if they are ulcerated with or without bleeding.
- *Gums*: through slight pressure applied with the tip of the tongue depressor, it is noted whether the gums appear pink and firm, edematous with or without redness, with or without bleeding, or if they bleed easily.
- *Teeth and prostheses*: whether the teeth are clean or not present, whether there are deposits or local concretions (interdental) or generalized, and, finally, when carious lesions are present.
- *Breath*: the operator assesses whether it is normal, if it is slightly to moderately bad, or if the patient emits a strong and bad smell.

The subject, on the basis of the score achieved on the test, is included in one of the three levels of oral health (normal oral health, mild dysfunction, severe dysfunction):

1. *Normal oral health* (from 8 to 10 points): the subject's oral health is normal, and the risk of pneumonia ab ingestis resulting from the ingestion of oral bacterial biofilms is low. The operator or the patient, the latter if autonomous, can continue the oral hygiene maneuvers as usually performed.
2. *Mild dysfunction* (from 11 to 14 points): moderate dysfunction of oral health, and the risk of pneumonia resulting from the ingestion of oral bacterial biofilms, is greater if no immediate precautions are taken. In this case, the operator and/or

caregiver or the patient, always if autonomous, must try to improve the oral situation, intensifying and performing the maneuvers of oral hygiene more accurately.
3. *Severe dysfunction* (from 15 to 24 points): severe oral health dysfunction and a greater risk of pneumonia *ab ingestis* caused by the ingestion of oral bacterial biofilms, which are highly rich in pathogenic species in people with poor oral hygiene. In this case, the operator, in addition to trying to improve the situation of the oral cavity, adhering to the indications concerning patients with moderate oral dysfunction, will have to contact the doctor.

In the case of the presence of oral mucosa alterations, it is necessary to carry out prevention, information, and education interventions and provide patients with strategies that can alleviate pain. In this sense, the following is suggested:

- Use ice cubes for the soothing effect sensation.
- Avoid spicy or acidic foods, and favor foods with a soft consistency.
- Proposal of low-salt foods.
- Frequently moisturize the mouth, and use fatty creams on the lips to prevent mucosal ulcerations.
- Take care of oral hygiene two or three times a day, with immediate treatment of infections (candida) if present and oral rinses with anesthetics.
- Pay the utmost care to the hygiene of the dental prosthesis, if present, at the end of each meal.
- Avoid fluoride toothpaste, which can irritate inflamed mucous membranes.
- Massage is performed daily, with a brush with soft bristles, on the gums, tongue, palate, and cheeks, to remove plaque, bacteria, and tartar, which can cause irritations, infections, and halitosis.

It is therefore essential that hygiene, oral rehydration, and the treatment of mucosal lesions are carried out constantly because their state is essential to allow chewing and taste function.

5.3.2 Communicating Food Choices

With respect to palliative feeding, it is important that the foods proposed fully meet the patient's desires. Respect for this basic criterion is not always easy to implement with patients who have communicative disabilities (Ball et al. 2012; Bonazzi and Mazio 2013; Flosi 2013). For the interlocutor, it is of fundamental importance to welcome the patient's wishes so that palliative feeding, which no longer has a nutritional meaning, can positively impact quality of life and is not experienced as a further source of external imposition and adaptation to an already burdensome reality. In this task, often difficult, augmentative alternative communication (AAC) is of considerable help. AAC is "any communication that replaces or increases verbal language [...] an area of clinical practice that seeks to compensate for the temporary or permanent disability of individuals with complex communication needs" (ASHA 2004). The adjective "augmentative," from the English *augmentative*, indicates that the communication methods used do not replace but increase those natural methods because the goal of AAC is the expansion of communication capabilities through all available channels and methods. The adjective "alternative" indicates that these communication methods are different and therefore alternative to those generally used. This term should not be misleading, as it does not aim to replace existing communication methods but rather to expand them. AAC is therefore an area of clinical practice that aims to reduce, contain, and compensate for communication disabilities, whether temporary or permanent, both on the expressive and receptive sides. This is achieved through the use, reinforcement, and expansion of existing methods; the enhancement of natural methods; and the introduction of special methods. The purpose of AAC intervention in a person with complex communication needs (CCN) is to support the development of communication skills in such a way that they can have full access to the possibilities of interacting with others, influencing the environment and fully participating in social life (Beukelman and Mirenda 2014). Those defined as "users with complex communication needs" are individuals who have communication problems associated with a wide range of physical, sensory, and environmental causes, which restrict and limit the ability to participate independently in society. People with complex communication needs and their communication partners can benefit from AAC both temporarily and permanently according to the definition of the Italian section of the *International Society for Augmentative and Alternative Communication* (ISAAC).

5.3.2.1 AAC Intervention

Historically, the first AAC assessment practices focused on identifying those individuals who possessed the necessary skills. The primary requirements are twofold: the ability to make or imitate sounds and the ability to understand and learn verbal language. This type of assessment was based on a model that established the prerequisites. Subsequently, the international literature has focused on a model that takes into account the needs of the person with a communication disorder, implementing an intervention in these needs. Current assessment procedures are based on a participatory model, according to which all people with severe disabilities can communicate. This perspective strengthens the model, whose key points are the opportunity to communicate and access communication.

The "participation-based model" (Beukelman and Mirenda 2005) is based on the following key principles (Fig. 5.9):

- Facilitate communication and participation in daily life activities and in society.
- Actively involve the subject and his or her living environment in the assessment, as they are the "best experts";
- Build a tailor-made project for the person, the family, and the context at the specific moment of their history.

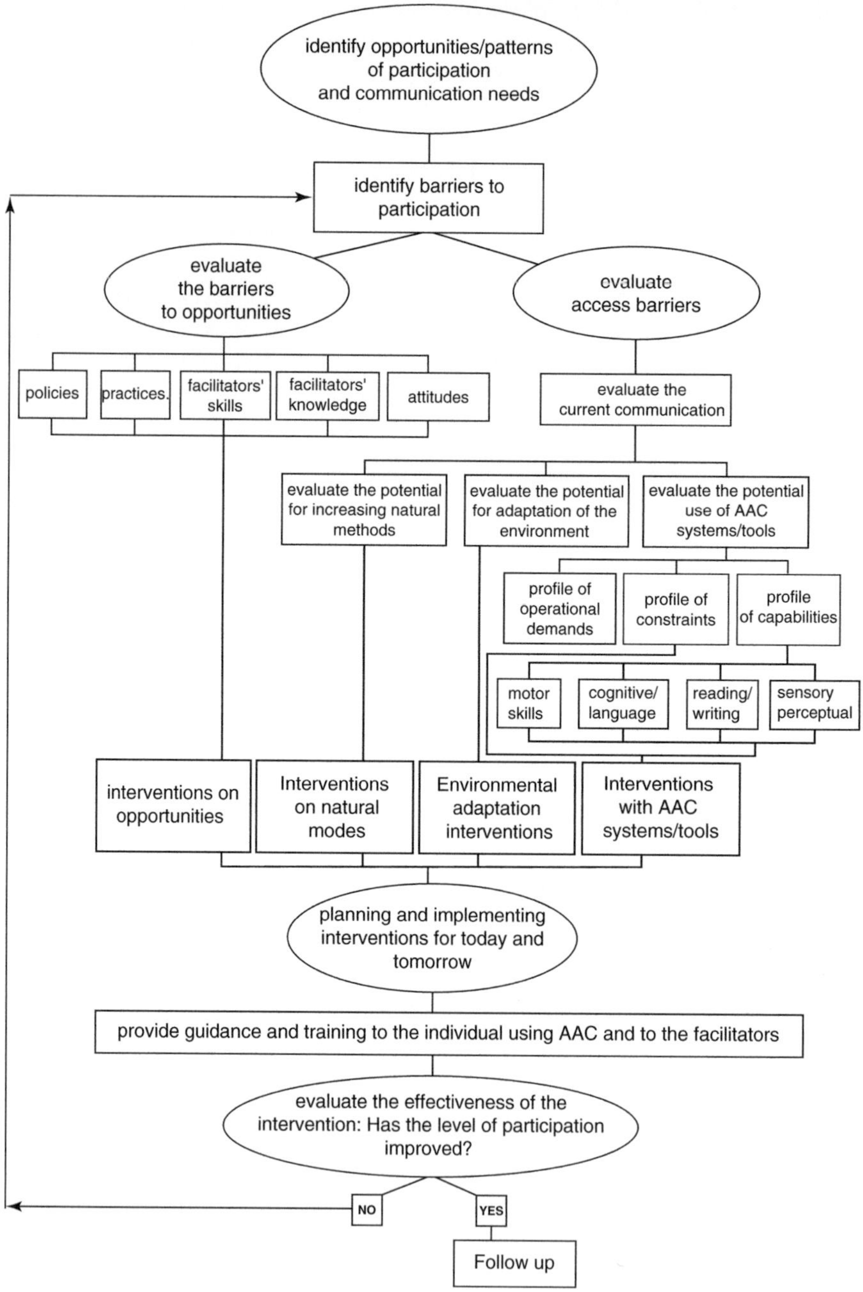

Fig. 5.9 Model of participation. (Source: Beukelman and Mirenda (2005))

This model focuses on identifying the opportunities for participation and the communication needs of the person. Barriers to participation are identified and evaluated, which can be of opportunity and/or access, and then the AAC intervention for the present and the future can be organized and planned through guidelines and training for the person with CCN and facilitators and/or caregivers (Beukelman and Light 2020).

5.3.2.2 Identifying Participation Methods and Communication Needs

It is important to identify the activities and people with whom the person with CCN interacts. In the case of a user who needs assistance during meals, we can identify various occasions, such as breakfast, lunch, and dinner, and various settings, such as the kitchen, the living room, and the bedroom, with different frequencies of use. At this point, it is also useful to consider the various people involved, such as husbands, wives, family members, caregivers, and strangers, as well as how often these people are involved and for how long. To determine the critical steps to intervene, it is necessary to understand how a subject without CCN participates in mealtime (Table 5.1).

5.3.2.3 Participation Barriers

By "barriers," we refer to the obstacles posed by people, which cannot be removed with a communication system or with an augmentative communication intervention. Barriers can be of *opportunity* or *access.*

The *opportunity barriers* are as follows:

- Political
- Of practice
- Of knowledge

Table 5.1 Example of a data collection grid for settings and partners for participation

Communication partners	Type of meal	Environments	Setting	Frequency
Husband/wife	Breakfast	Kitchen	2 people	Every day
Parent	Lunch	Living room	More people	2/3 times a week
Child	Dinner	Bedroom	Noisy environment	Once a week
Other family member	Small quantity administration	Restaurant	Quiet environment	Every 15 days
Caregiver				Occasionally
Friends				
Helpers				
Medical staff				
Strangers				

Source: adapted from Beukelman et al. (2007)

- Of skills
- Of attitude

Political barriers are determined by legislative or administrative provisions of a person's living environment with a BCC in the case of hospitals or residential or rehabilitative centers. They can also be unwritten provisions, in the case of a family context, in which they are still set by the decision-maker, for example, a spouse or a support administrator. An example of a possible political barrier is the inability to access the prescription of a personal computer for a pathology or disability different from what is regulated.

Practice or praxis barriers are procedures that have become routine in a specific context, without any real written rules and especially evidence related to these practices. An example is the low use of AAC with BCC users because, by practice, the use of this approach is implemented as a *last resort.*

Knowledge barriers refer to the absence or lack of information that leads the caregiver, family member, or other person to limit the participation of the person with BCC in rehabilitative activities. An example of this is the lack of knowledge about the possibility of organizing a CAA intervention.

Skill barriers materialize when, even with the necessary and adequate information, those who take care of the person with BCC have difficulty putting into practice what they have learned and therefore need further practice to remove the obstacles that limit their communicative competence.

Attitude or behavior barriers are obstacles consisting of limiting and negative attitudes on the part of anyone interacting with the person with BCC, who, in this way, is limited in his/her communicative opportunities.

Opportunity barriers are not always surmountable, and in some cases, they are not surmountable in the short term when, for example, a regulation or an administrative rule must be modified (Light 2007). Augmentative communication interventions must take into maximum consideration such barriers and try to overcome them through information and the active involvement of all interested parties. In some situations, such as for knowledge or skill barriers, these can be broken down through information and practice. In other cases, such as political barriers, it is necessary to acknowledge them and find solutions that can overcome the barrier even without the possibility of modifying it immediately. A great example of an intervention aimed at overcoming practice barriers is represented by the Guidelines for Meeting the Communication Needs of Person with Severe Disabilities (1992), developed by the National Committee for the Communication Needs of Persons with Severe Disabilities. The text

Box 5.5 Charter of Rights to Communication
All persons, regardless of their degree of disability, have the fundamental right to influence, through communication, the conditions of their own existence. In addition to this basic right, the following specific rights must be guaranteed:

1. The right to request objects, actions, and people and to express preferences and feelings.
2. The right to choose between different alternatives.
3. The right to refuse unwanted objects, situations, and actions and not to accept all the choices proposed.
4. The right to ask for and receive attention and to have exchanges with other people.
5. The right to request information about objects, people, situations or facts of interest.
6. The right to activate all interventions that make it possible for them to communicate messages, in any way and in the most effective manner, regardless of the degree of disability.
7. The right to have their communicative act recognized anyway and to receive a response even if it is not possible to satisfy the request.
8. The right to have access at any time to every need for augmentative alternative communication assistance facilitates and improves communication and the right to always have it updated and in good working conditions.
9. The right to participate as a communication partner, with the same rights as any other person, in the contexts, interactions and opportunities of everyday life.
10. The right to be informed about people, things and facts related to one's living environment.
11. The right to receive information to participate in discussions that take place in the living environment, respecting the dignity of the person with disabilities.
12. The right to receive messages in a comprehensible and culturally and linguistically appropriate manner.

Source: National Committee for the Communication Needs of Persons with Severe Disabilities, 1992 (Italian translation by ISAAC Italy).

aims to form shared guidelines of CAA interventions and contains the Charter of rights to communication (Box 5.5).

The *access barriers* are the limitations in abilities, resources, and attitudes of people who use, or could use, augmentative communication:

- Physical and/or motor barriers
- Cognitive barriers
- Literacy barriers
- Visual and/or auditory barriers

Physical and/or motor barriers: In relation to these barriers, it is important to have the necessary motor control to use alternative access for communication, such as direct selection through pointing or gaze or mediated selection through the use of technological tools that require movement to initiate the choice.

Cognitive barriers: These barriers can include some aspects of cognitive-communicative development that are very relevant for AAC: awareness, communicative intentionality, knowledge of the world, memory, symbolic representation, and metacognitive abilities (Rowland and Schweigert 2003). Other authors (Wilkinson and Jagaroo 2004) also consider some visual-perceptive abilities to be important.

Literacy barriers: Literacy skills substantially include the ability to read, spell, and write.

Visual and/or auditory barriers: Visual barriers can affect the type, size, spacing, positioning, and colors of symbols and characters; auditory barriers affect the types of linguistic input and output to be adapted to the person with SCC.

Importantly, access barriers and related abilities should be evaluated to the extent that they influence the communication of the person with SCC, which is therefore relevant to AAC intervention (Yorkston and Karlan 1986). Beyond access barriers, it is necessary to verify the methods currently used by the person to communicate and the effectiveness of such communication.

5.3.2.4 Interventions for the Natural and Adaptive Modes of the Environment

Within the scope of augmentative communication, when we talk about "natural modes," we refer to language, vocalization, and the use of gestures or other codes for communicative purposes:

- Facial expressions
- Head movements
- Body movements
- Vocalizations, attempts at speech/words
- Conventional or nonconventional gestures
- Pantomime
- Sign languages
- Finger spelling

Language, if present, is evaluated for its communicative potential on the basis of intelligibility and the user's effort to produce it. It is also useful for evaluating the possibility of *supplemented intelligibility*, that is, the extent to which the listener can understand the speaker if the statement is integrated with contextual information such as the topic, the first letters of words, and possibly gestures (Hanson et al. 2004). The intervention in these modes will therefore be calibrated not to the intelligibility of the language itself but to the different conditions in which it is used. If it is too strenuous or inadvisable for the user to use language during mealtime, it is preferable to accompany other natural augmentative modes to facilitate the communication of needs and desires but also as an exchange of information, knowledge, ideas, and feelings, therefore serving as a tool of social closeness.

These natural modes can be organized according to the needs and motor and cognitive skills of the user to define a multimodal communication system that exploits residual abilities and uses them for communicative purposes. It will be useful to organize them so that, with the use of a specific gesture or vocalization, one and only one meaning corresponds; or again, one can use the movement of the head or of another part of the body to identify the "yes" and the "no." Finally, another option involves evaluating the possibility of indicating with the look, the hand, the finger, or other body districts.

The environment can be modified in an attempt to eliminate any barrier that may interfere with communication, such as a noisy environment, or in case of the need for larger spaces to place the caregiver in front of the user, to facilitate communication, or again, in case of necessary adaptations to reposition any aids useful for communication.

5.3.2.5 Interventions with AAC Systems and Aids

The evaluation of current communication modes, specific communication needs, and access and opportunity barriers leads to organizing a possible use of AAC tools, chosen among those available, which are suitable for the person's immediate needs, taking into account current linguistic, motor, cognitive, and sensory abilities, as well as the limits and any opportunity barriers not yet overcome (Flosi and Pieri 2016). This system must be accurate and efficient but not tiring. An *accurate* system is one that the person can use to produce messages with the minimum number of interruptions and errors. An *efficient* system is one that avoids long periods of practice or training by the person and communication partners. A *non-tiring* system allows the AAC user to communicate for as long as necessary without becoming tired and without becoming less precise and efficient.

5.3.2.6 Symbols

A symbol is something that represents or stands for something else (Vanderheiden and Yoder 1986), which is called its "referent." Symbols are often classified on the basis of their iconicity, that is, on the association the person establishes between a symbol and its referent (Schlosser 2003).

To understand what type of symbols to use, even when combined, for a user with BCC, the symbols must be distinguished:

- Depending on the *iconicity*: a symbol can be *transparent,* and therefore, the shape, movement, or function of the referent is represented such that the meaning of the symbol can be readily identified even in the absence of the referent

(Fuller and Lloyd 1991). An example can be the drawing or photo of a spoon. An *opaque* symbol is instead a written word: in continuity with the previous example, the written word "spoon" is an opaque symbol, as there is no perceptible relationship between the symbol and referent.

- Between *aided* and *unaided*: *aided* symbols (with aid) require some type of external support to the person for production, whereas *unaided* symbols (without aid) do not require an external device (Lloyd and Fuller 1986). Examples of *aided* symbols include tangible objects (the spoon) and pictographic symbols (the image of the spoon); examples of *unaided* symbols include facial expressions, gestures, vocalizations, and words.

5.3.2.7 Selection Techniques

Selection techniques constitute the method by which the person using AAC selects or identifies an item to communicate. These are the main options:

- *Direct selection*: through which the person directly indicates the desired item with the finger or by touching it, applying pressure, through a pointer, or even with the gaze, through the indication (*pointing*) of the eyes.
- *Scanning selection*: this is used in case of the user's inability to choose an item directly. This often occurs due to a lack of motor control. In these situations, it is the communication partner of the person with the BCC, or an electronic system, that presents the items. The user with the BCC must wait for the partner or the electronic aid to scan through the items until they reach the desired one. At this point, the person with the BCC signals, in the preselected and previously agreed-upon way, that the item has been identified. The scan can occur in different ways, for example, *circular*, in the case of items drawn as on a clock; *linear* for rows, in the case of scanning the items one after another horizontally; for *columns*, in the case of vertical scanning; and *block*, when referring to various groups of items (once the block is chosen, a further scan is carried out within the block itself to find the preselected item). The cognitive effort in scanning selection is greater than that required in direct selection.

5.3.3 *Low-Technology Aids* (Low-Tech)

Low-technology aids are those that rely on the use of pen and paper and alert systems, such as call bells, writing systems, and tables. Some are listed below:

- The *communication boards* are aids built with paper, plastic, plexiglass, etc. and contain symbols in the form of images or pictograms and/or letters, numbers, words, and phrases. They are usually *fixed displays*, also called "static." However, it is possible to attach and detach items on and from the boards if necessary for the AAC user. The number of items is limited and may depend on the user's visual, tactile, cognitive, and motor abilities.

With any display based on visual or auditory options, the number of items is the result of a compromise between the number of symbols necessary for the person, the format of the symbols themselves and the display, and the spacing and arrangement of the items. It is also necessary to consider the color of the display background and the items present, to guarantee that the user has the greatest possibility of discrimination.

For the *icons*, if there are many, it may be preferable to use them in black and white because they are less fatiguing and more functional and allow you to use a glance, facilitating the shift from one symbol to another and therefore better maintaining attention even for persons with a visual problem. On the other hand, color can be better used if there is a need to stimulate attention (Costantino 2012).

For the *type of font*, highly readable fonts, such as OpenDyslexic and dyslexie and easyreading are free, which are free fonts, or Sylexiad and EasyReading, which are instead paid, can be used.

These findings have been evaluated by various studies on dyslexia; however for more recent fonts as TestMe, Baincoenero and Lexie Readable no studies are available. From the results of various studies on fonts, it appears that there is not one that, a priori, is better for readability than traditional fonts used for this purpose, such as Helvetica, Arial, and Verdana, while some studies also report the Georgia font. To facilitate readability, in addition to font, the importance of formatting is highlighted; therefore, the spacing between letters and letters in words, between words, and between lines needs to be considered and adjusted. The studies mainly concern fonts with sizes between 10 and 16, those typical of the text written in the majority of books, whereas in alphabetic tables, larger characters are predominantly used.

For each sentence, in addition to formatting, it is important to evaluate its length and complexity: taking inspiration from the controlled writing studies of De Mauro and Piemontese, it is advisable to use short and linear sentences without coordinate and subordinate clauses and with the entire core of meaning expressed in one line.

It is therefore necessary to evaluate the orientation of the display, that is, its inclination with respect to the floor and therefore the suitable positioning for the person with BCC, in relation to his visual and motor abilities.

The user will be able to use these aids alone, by indication of gaze or with the mediation of the communicative partner, who will perform the scan by reading and/or indicating each item, according to the scanning method provided and with a method agreed upon in advance. A nod of the head, a movement of the eyes, a vocalization, or others may indicate consent at the time of presentation of the desired item.

- The *list tables* are lists of words on paper/cardboard/transparent support, which the person with BCC can indicate directly or through scanning assisted by the communication partner (Table 5.2).
- The *alphabetical tables* are paper or plastic displays that use graphemes, words, phrases, and numbers. Tables can be arranged in "querty" order, such as the computer keyboard, or in alphabetical order.

Table 5.2 Example of a choice list

I need:	First course
Pause	• Pasta with ragout
Drink	• Rice and peas
Less	• Lasagna
Slower	• Cannelloni

- The *picture/icon boards* are paper, cardboard, plastic, or other material supports that allow for the use of various types of images to support communication. There are various types of boards: for example, for the meal or the administration of boluses, a so-called theme table could be constructed, which includes everything that can be useful in that context for the user, such as inserting the possibility of giving indications on what is preferred and expressing comments. Iconographic symbols are not commonly used by adults, but if they are used, black and white symbols are preferred.
- The *placemats* are paper or plastic supports with icons regarding the possibility of making requests, expressing choices and making comments at mealtime.
- *E-TRAN* is a name coming from the contraction of the English phrase *eye transfer* or "exchange with the gaze" (E-TRAN). It is usually made up of a transparent panel on which symbols, letters, or numbers are written, imprinted or attached. The materials normally used for panels are plexiglass and Lexan, which are relatively resistant to scratches, but a sheet of glossy paper, which is rollable, can also be used. Its size varies depending on the user and his motor and visual abilities; usually, the maximum format is approximately 40 × 50 cm.

The transparent panel is placed between the user and the communication partner: when the former looks at an item on the panel, the latter, from the opposite side, can see where the gaze is directed and the element that is indicated (Fig. 5.1). There are two modes of using this device: one can keep the E-TRAN board still and the user searches for the desired item, or the communication partner can move the E-TRAN in front of the user's eyes until he stops it at the chosen item (Fig. 5.10).

Understanding, as a rule, is quite rapid, as are communication exchanges.

In case of incorrect interpretation or error, there may be an item to indicate it, and it will be useful to place a symbol for the end of the word and a symbol for the question sentence. You can then also add the words "yes" and "no."

- The *communicative passport* is a tool introduced and described in the 1990s by Sally Millar in the Anglo-Saxon context; it is useful for understanding all the characteristics of the person with BCC to those who will have a role of care or assistance to put the latter in a position to best welcome the person. It can be built in paper or digital form, reporting all the important information about the person and how they communicate (Millar and Aitken 2003). The passport therefore reports the natural and special augmentative modes employed by the user and how to manage them, in addition to all the information related to correct care during feeding.

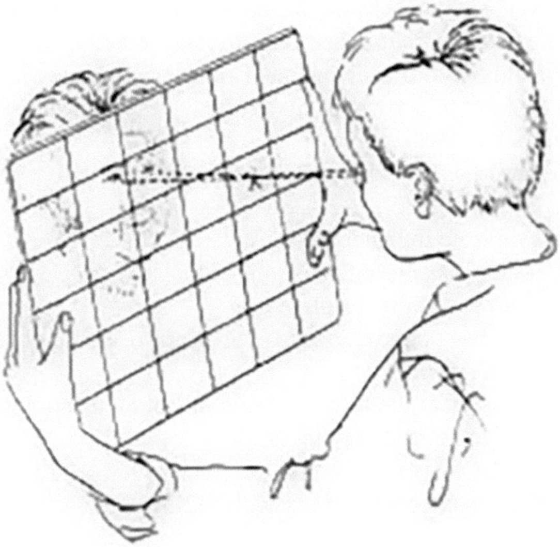

Fig. 5.10 Example of using the E-TRAN. (Drawing by Cecilia Amitrano)

5.3.3.1 High-Technology Aids (High-Tech)

Any device created for AAC, such as "alphabetical and symbolic communicators," software, or the most recent apps, which are also available for PCs, tablets, and smartphones, has a great potential and large possibilities of use: much depends on the digital skills of the user with the BCC and the possible caregiver (Koch Fager et al. 2019).

Through dedicated applications, it will be possible to use the same images, letters, or words of the paper tables, with the possibility of a dynamic display that allows, for example, opening a set of symbols linked to the chosen item, thus expanding and accelerating the communicative exchange. In addition to what has already been illustrated about the characteristics of the items, adjusting the brightness that can make the display more adaptable to the user and the environments in which the use of such tools takes place is important.

The use of the synthesized voice output of type *text-to-speech* (TTS) allows the voice to be converted into the written text, even if the synthesized voice is not always well understood and accepted by the user and, sometimes, listening training should therefore be considered.

5.3.4 The Communicative Partners

The communicative partners are people who have social, educational, and care relationships with AAC users. Family members, friends, colleagues, teachers, health professionals, assistants, and other similar figures are all communicative partners who can be identified as "facilitators," according to the definition of Cumley and Beukelman (1992). Communication is a dynamic and interactive process in which communicative partners continuously influence each other, reciprocally, during the entire course of their interaction (Mcnaughton and Light

1989). The success of the communicative exchange depends on all the people who take part in it. It is therefore important that the AAC intervention is addressed not only to the user but also to the facilitators, according to the definition of ASHA for which "AAC also refers to the sole adjustments in the behaviors of the interlocutors."

In particular, communicative partners:

- Dominate the interaction
- Mainly ask closed questions (which only expect "yes" or "no" as an answer)
- Hold the communicative turn
- Give few opportunities to AAC users to initiate and respond during the interaction
- Often interrupt
- Focus their attention on communication technologies or techniques, rather than AAC users or their messages

On the other hand, users with BCC:

- Assume passive roles
- Use limited communication functions
- Use limited linguistic forms

Some facilitators succeed in their task without specific preparation; others need to be trained to positively support interaction with the AAC user (Kent-Walsh and Mcnaughton 2005). It is therefore useful to provide learning programs for facilitators that also provide the necessary skills to effectively support interaction, in addition to teaching the operation of the user's communication system AAC and illustrating the various environmental adjustments for any aid (positioning, maintenance, care, implementation, etc.).

References

Almomani F, Brown C, Williams KB. The effect of an oral health promotion program for people with psychiatric disabilities. Psychiatr Rehabil J. 2006;29(4):274–81.

American Speech-Language- Hearing Association – Special Interest Division 12: Augmentative and Alternative Communication – Roles and Responsibility of speech-language pathologist with respect to Augmentative and Alternative Communication. Technical Report – ASHA Supplement, vol. 24 - Ruoli e responsabilità del Logopedista rispetto alla Comunicazione Aumentativa ed Alternativa: Relazione tecnica - Traduzione italiana a cura di ISAAC Italy in: Argomenti di Comunicazione Aumentativa e Alternativa, 12, 2015. 2004.

Amitrano A. Dysphagia as mourning. Italian Palliative Care J. 2019;21(1):46–50.

Aremyr G. Live life forgetful. Activation of Alzheimer's patients. Oslo: Kommunefor-laget; 1993.

Asadoorian J, Locker D. The impact of quality assurance programming: a comparison of two Canadian dental hygienist programs. J Dent Educ. 2006;70(9):965–71.

Australian Government Department of Social Services. Better Oral health in residential care. Staff portfolio: education and training program. Adelaide: SA Dental Service; 2009. https://dhaa.info/common/Uploaded%20files/OHPPH/StaffPortfolio.pdf.

Ball LJ, Fager S, Fried-Oken M. Augmentative and alternative communication for people with progressive neurological disease. Phys Med Rehabil Clin N Am. 2012;23(3):689–99.

Bartlett JG, Gorbach SL, Finegold SM. The bacteriology of aspiration pneumonia. Am J Med. 1974;56(2):202–7. https://doi.org/10.1016/0002-9343(74)90598-1.

Bassim CW, Gibson G, Ward T, Paphides BM, Denucci DJ. Modification of the risk of mortality from pneumonia with oral hygiene care. J Am Geriatr Soc. 2008;56(9):1601–7. https://doi.org/10.1111/j.1532-5415.2008.01825.x.

Beukelman D, Light J. Augmentative and alternative communication for children and adults. 5th ed. Baltimore: Paul H. Brookes; 2020.

Beukelman D, Mirenda P. Augmentative and alternative communication for children and adults. 3rd ed. Baltimore: Paul H. Brookes; 2005.

Beukelman D, Mirenda P. Manual of augmentative and alternative communication. Interventions for children and adults with complex communication needs. Trento: Erickson; 2014.

Beukelman D, Garrett K, Yorkston K. Augmentative communication strategies for adults with acute or chronic medical condition. Baltimore: Paul H. Brookes; 2007.

Bonazzi C, Amitrano A. The counselling. In: Ruoppolo G, Schindler A, Amitrano A, Genovese E, editors. Manual of phoniatrics and speech therapy. Roma: Society Editrice Universo; 2012.

Bonazzi C, Mazio G. Augmentative and alternative communication in motor speech disorders. In: Ruoppolo G, Amitrano A, editors. Dysarthria. Can we do more? Torino: Omega Edizioni; 2013.

Borasio GD. Knowing how to die: what we can do, how to prepare. Torino: Bollati Boringhieri; 2015.

Bundesärztekammer. Principles of the Federal Medical Association for medical end-of-life care. Deutsches Arzteblatt. 2004;51:A 1298 ss. as well as cviii 2011, p. A346.

Chalmers JM, Carter KD, Spencer AJ. Caries incidence and increments in community-living older adults with and without dementia. Gerodontology. 2002;19(2):80–94.

Corvo P, Fassino G. When food becomes wellness: nutrition and quality of life. Milano: Franco Angeli; 2015.

Costantino MA. Building books and stories with the AAC. Trento: Erickson; 2012.

Cumley G, Beukelman D. Roles and responsibilities of facilitators in augmentative and alternative communication. Semin Speech Lang. 1992;13(2):111–8.

Eilers J, Berger AM, Petersen MC. Development, testing, and application of the oral assessment guide. Oncol Nurs Forum. 1988;15(3):325–30.

Fischler C. The omnivore, the pleasure of eating in history and science. Milano: Mondadori; 1990.

Flosi C. Augmentative alternative communication with adult people in the neurological field. Genova: GEDI Gruppo Editoriale; 2013.

Flosi C, Pieri M. Is it appropriate? Tools for the evaluation of applications in support of the augmentative alternative communication of people with complex communication needs. Genova: GEDI Gruppo Editoriale; 2016.

Fuller D, Lloyd L. Toward a common usage of iconicity terminology. Augment Altern Commun. 1991;7(3):215–20.

Hanson E, Yorkston K, Beukelman D. Speech supplementation techniques for dysarthria: a systematic review. J Med Speech Lang Pathol. 2004;12(2):9–29.

Hartzband P, Groopman J. Keeping the patient in the equation-humanism and health care reform. N Engl J Med. 2009;361(6):554–5.

Kelly K, Cumming S, Kenny B, Smith-Merry J, Bogaardt H. Getting comfortable with "comfort feeding": an exploration of legal and ethical aspects of the Australian speech-language pathologist's role in palliative dysphagia care. Int J Speech Lang Pathol. 2018;20(3):371–9. https://doi.org/10.1080/17549507.2018.1448895.

Kent-Walsh J, Mcnaughton O. Communication partner instruction in AAC: present practices and future directions. Augment Altern Commun. 2005;21(3):195–204.

Koch Fager S, Fried-Oken M, Jakobs T, Beukelman DR. New and emerging access technologies for adults with complex communication needs and severe motor impairments: state of the science. Augment Altern Commun. 2019;35(1):13–25. https://doi.org/10.1080/07434618.2018.1556730.

Light J. Toward a definition of communicative competence for individuals using augmentative and alternative communication systems. Augment Altern Commun. 2007;5(2):137–44.

Lloyd L, Fuller D. Toward an augmentative and alternative communication symbol taxonomy: a proposed superordinate classification. Augment Altern Commun. 1986;2(4):165–71.

Lux J. Review of the Oral disease. Systemic disease link. Part 1: heart disease, diabetes. Can J Dent Hyg. 2006;40(6):288–342.

Marik PE. Aspiration pneumonitis and aspiration pneumonia. N Engl J Med. 2001;344(9):665–71.

Martins S, Castro AS. Speech therapy in palliative care-Portuguese perspective. J Palliat Med. 2017;20(1):7.

Mcnaughton D, Light J. Teaching facilitators to support the communication skills of an adult with severe cognitive disabilities: a case study. Augment Altern Commun. 1989;5(1):35–41.

Mercadante S, Ripamonti C. Medicine and palliative care in oncology. Clinical, care and organizational aspects. Milan: Masson; 2002.

Millar S, Aitken S. Personal communication passports: guidelines for good practice. Edinburgh: CALL Centre; 2003.

O'Reilly AC, Walshe M. Perspectives on the role of the speech and language therapist in palliative care: an international survey. Palliat Med. 2015;29(8):756–61.

Petersen PE, Bourgeois D, Ogawa H, Estupinan-Day S, Ndiaye C. The global burden of oral diseases and risks to oral health. Bull World Health Organ. 2005;83(9):661–9.

Portney LG, Watkins MP. Foundations of clinical research. Applications to practice. Upper Saddle River: Prentice Hall; 2007.

Prandi C. Nursing in palliative care. Milan: Edra; 2015.

Prendergast V, Kleiman C, King M. The Bedside Oral Exam and the Barrow Oral Care Protocol: translating evidence-based oral care into practice. Intensive Crit Care Nurs. 2013;29(5):282–90. https://doi.org/10.1016/j.iccn.2013.04.001.

Provinciali L, Carlini G, Tarquini D, Defanti CA, Veronese S, Pucci E. Need for palliative care for neurological diseases. Neurol Sci. 2016;37(10):1581–7. https://doi.org/10.1007/s10072-016-2614-x.

Quagliarello V, Ginter S, Han L, Van Ness P, Allore H, Tinetti M. Modifiable risk factors for nursing home-acquired pneumonia. Clin Infect Dis. 2005;40(1):1–6. https://doi.org/10.1086/426023.

Rapley M. Quality of life research. A critical introduction. London: SAGE; 2003.

Rowland C, Schweigert P. Cognitive skills and IIC. In: Light J, Beukelman D, Reichle J, editors. Communicative competence for individuals who use IIC: from research to effective practice. Baltimore: Paul H. Brookes; 2003. p. 241–75.

Scalmani L.B, et al. Comparison ratings of pureed versus molded fruits: preliminary results, "Dysphagia". 2000;15(1) pp.2–5.

Scannapieco FA, Bush RB, Paju S. Associations between periodontal disease and risk for atherosclerosis, cardiovascular disease, and stroke. A systematic review. Ann Periodontol. 2003;8(1):38–53. https://doi.org/10.1902/annals.2003.8.1.38.

Schlosser R. Selecting graphic symbols for an initial request lexicon. In: Schlosser R, editor. The efficacy of augmentative and alternative communication: toward evidence-based practice. New York: Elsevier; 2003. p. 347–402.

Sheiham A. Oral health, general health and quality of life. Bull World Health Organ. 2005;83(9):644.

Sjögren P, Nilsson E, Forsell M, Johansson O, Hoogstraate J. A systematic review of the preventive effect of oral hygiene on pneumonia and respiratory tract infection in elderly people in hospitals and nursing homes: effect estimates and methodological quality of randomized controlled trials. J Am Geriatr Soc. 2008;56(11):2124–30. https://doi.org/10.1111/j.1532-5415.2008.01926.x.

Son YG, Shin J, Ryu HG. Pneumonitis and pneumonia after aspiration. J Dent Anesth Pain Med. 2017;17(1):1–12.

Sumi Y, Nakamura Y, Michiwaki Y. Development of a systematic oral care program for frail elderly persons. Spec Care Dentist. 2002;22(4):151–5. https://doi.org/10.1111/j.1754-4505.2002.tb01180.x.

Sumi Y, Miura H, Michiwaki Y, Nagaosa S, Nagaya M. Colonization of dental plaque by respiratory pathogens in dependent elderly. Arch Gerontol Geriatr. 2007;44(2):119–24. https://doi.org/10.1016/j.archger.2006.04.004.

Vanderheiden G, Yoder D. Overview. In: Blackstone S, editor. Augmentative communication: an introduction. Rockville: American Speech-Language-Hearing Association; 1986. p. 1–28.

Vucea V, Keller HH, Morrison JM, Duizer LM, Duncan AM, Carrier N, Lengyel CO, Slaughter SE, Steele CM. Modified texture food use is associated with malnutrition in long term care: an analysis of Making the Most of Mealtimes (M3) Project. J Nutr Health Aging. 2018;22(8):916–22. https://doi.org/10.1007/s12603-018-1016-6.

Watt RG. Strategies and approaches in oral disease prevention and health promotion. Bull World Health Organ. 2005;83(9):711–8.

Weyant RJ, Jones JA, Hobbins M, Niessen LC, Adelson R, Rhyne RR. Oral health status of a long-term-care, veteran population. Community Dent Oral Epidemiol. 1993;21(4):227–33. https://doi.org/10.1111/j.1600-0528.1993.tb00762.x.

Wilkinson K, Jagaroo V. Contribution of principles of visual cognitive science to AAC system display design. Augment Altern Commun. 2004;20(3):123–6.

Yorkston K, Karlan G. Assessment procedures. In: Blackstone S, editor. Augmentative communication: an introduction. Rockville, MD: American Speech-Language-Hearing Association; 1986. p. 163–96.

Zucconi A, Howell P. Health promotion: a global approach for the Well-being of the individual and society. Molfetta: La meridiana; 2003.

Websites

www.communicationpassports.org.uk.

www.aiditalia.org.

INRAN. www.crea.gov.it. 2003.

Appendix

A. Amitrano, *Dysphagia and Nutrition*,
https://doi.org/10.1007/978-3-031-77449-2

Form A

Dysphagia risk score 2 (DRS 2)

By Antonio Amitrano, Giulia Rossi and Francesca Romana Pezzella

Last Name...First Name..

Born on..Sex M ❑F ❑ NIHSS Scale ....

Check the box corresponding to the answer			Comment
Patient's age ***Patient ≥ 80 years?***	yes ❑ no ❑	1 0	
Level of consciousness ***Patient alert?***	yes ❑ no ❑	0 1	
Cough test ***Patient able to cough voluntarily?***	yes ❑ no ❑	0 3	
Water test ***Patient able to drink a glass of water without coughing?***	yes ❑ no ❑	0 3	
After drinking the glass of water, voice has changed?	yes ❑ no ❑	3 0	
Drooling?	yes ❑ no ❑	0.5 0	
Does he/she spit out saliva independently?	yes ❑ no ❑	3 0	
Shortness of breath?	yes ❑ no ❑	2 0	
TOTAL			

Risk rating	Absent Total = 0	Low 0.5 ≤ total = 3	Medium 3.5 ≤ total = 5	High Total ≥ 5.5

Administrator: ______________________		Date: ______________
Speech therapy evaluation requested	Fail **YES**	Pass **NO**

Form B

Meal observation grid

By Antonio Amitrano and Valentina Crinelli.

- **Observed subjects**

Surname: ____________________

Name: ______________________

Date of observation: ______________________

Date of onset of pathological event: ______________________

- **Aetiology**

☐Brainstem stroke

☐Cerebral stroke

☐Cerebellar stroke

☐Head trauma

☐Multiple sclerosis

☐Amyotrophic lateral sclerosis

☐Neoplasia

☐Parkinson's Disease

☐Other

- **Check list**

1. The patient is lying in bed during the meal:
   yes ☐ no ☐
2. The patient is seated:
   ☐ in a wheelchair
   ☐ on a chair
   ☐ on the bed
3. During the meal, a caregiver is present:
   yes ☐ no ☐
4. The patient is self-sufficient in eating:
   yes ☐ no ☐
5. The patient has the ability to start the meal independently:
   yes ☐ no ☐

6. The patient is able to use cutlery properly:
   yes ☐ no ☐
7. The patient spills food on him/herself:
   yes ☐ no ☐
8. The patient uses the napkin appropriately:
   yes ☐ no ☐
9. The patient starts eating only if prompted:
   yes ☐ no ☐
10. The patient refuses food:
    yes ☐no ☐
11. The consistency of the food is as follows:

    ☐ solid

    ☐ semisolid

    ☐ liquid

    ☐ semiliquid

    ☐ dual consistency

12. The patient used a dental prosthesis:
    yes ☐no ☐
13. The patient is able to chew:
    yes ☐no ☐
14. The patient swallows without chewing:
    yes ☐ no ☐
15. The patient keeps her lips closed during chewing:
    yes ☐ no ☐
16. There is food leakage from the mouth during chewing:

    yes ☐ no ☐
17. Presents drooling:
    yes ☐ no ☐
18. There is food leakage from the nose:
    yes ☐ no ☐
19. Residues after chewing:

    yes ☐ no ☐

If yes:

☐ on the lips

☐ in the mouth

20. Food residues remaining on the spoon (or fork):

    yes ☐ no ☐

21. The patient talks while eating:
    yes ❑ no ❑
22. The patient watches television while eating:
    yes ❑ no ❑
23. The patient continuously looks around:
    yes ❑ no ❑
24. The patient is constantly distracted by people in the room:

    yes ❑ no ❑

25. Repeatedly gets up from the chair:
    yes ❑ no ❑
26. The patient continuously changes posture:
    yes ❑ no ❑
27. The patient cries:
    yes ❑ no ❑
28. The patient takes long pauses between bites:
    yes ❑ no ❑
29. The patient takes food from the plate, ignoring what is on his/her left or right side:

    yes ❑ no ❑

30. The liquid intake is as follows:

    ❑ glass

    ❑ cup

    ❑ spoon

    ❑straw

    ❑ NG tube

    ❑ PEG

31. The patient drinks in small sips:
    yes ❑ no ❑
32. Drinks continuously:
    yes ❑ no ❑
33. Episodes of coughing/during food intake:

    yes ❑ no ❑

If yes, it occurs with:

☐ Solid foods

☐ semisolid foods

☐liquids

☐ semiliquids

☐ dual consistency

The cough is as follows:

☐violent

☐ violent with food coming out

☐raclage

34. After and during a meal, the voice is as follows:

☐ normal

☐ hoarse

☐ low

☐ veiled

☐ blown

☐ choked

☐ gurgling

☐ damp

☐ voiceless

35. The patient uses a particular head position:

yes ☐ no ☐

If yes:

☐ the head is flexed forward

☐ the head is flexed sideways

☐ the head is rotated

☐ the head is extended

36. The patient eats the first course:

Yes ☐ no ☐

If yes, completely:

yes ☐ no ☐

37. The patient eats the second course:

yes ☐ no ☐

If yes, completely:

yes ☐ no ☐

38. The patient eats the side dish:
    yes ☐ no ☐

    If yes, completely:
    yes ☐ no ☐

39. The patient eats fruit:

    yes ☐ no ☐

    If yes, completely:

    yes ☐ no ☐

40. The patient takes medication orally during the meal:

    Yes ☐ no ☐

    If yes, what type:

    ☐Capsule

    ☐tablets

    ☐ effervescent tablets

    ☐ lozenges

    ☐ gel

    ☐ drops

    ☐powders

    ☐ syrups

    They cause episodes of coughing:

    Yes ☐ no ☐

41. Meal time duration (*indicate the time*): ____________________________

Form C

Mealtime Assessment Tool (MAT) By Antonio Amitrano and Giulia Rossi.

Patient: ________________ Age: _______ Date: ____________ Meal: Breakfast Lunch Dinner

Who is completing the form: ____________________________________ Date: ___________

1. Does the patient actively participate during the meal?

Always 5	Almost always 4	Sometimes 3	Almost never 2	Never 1	N/A 0

2. Is the patient seated during the meal?

Always 5	Almost always 4	Sometimes 3	Almost never 2	Never 1	N/A 0

3. Are tablet, computer and television off during the meal?

Always 5	Almost always 4	Sometimes 3	Almost never 2	Never 1	N/A 0

4. Can the patient eat autonomously?

Always 5	Almost always 4	Sometimes 3	Almost never 2	Never 1	N/A 0

5. Does the patient drink during the meal?

Always 5	Almost always 4	Sometimes 3	Almost never 2	Never 1	N/A 0

6. Does the patient eat the complete meal?

Always 5	Almost always 4	Sometimes 3	Almost never 2	Never 1	N/A 0

7. Does the patient eat in silence?

Always 5	Almost always 4	Sometimes 3	Almost never 2	Never 1	N/A 0

8. Does the patient eat without coughing?

Always 5	Almost always 4	Sometimes 3	Almost never 2	Never 1	N/A 0

9. Does the patient's voice change before and after the meal?

Always 5	Almost always 4	Sometimes 3	Almost never 2	Never 1	N/A 0

10. Are the patient's lips clean from food residues after chewing?

Always 5	Almost always 4	Sometimes 3	Almost never 2	Never 1	N/A 0

11. Is the tongue clean from food residues after chewing?

Always 5	Almost always 4	Sometimes 3	Almost never 2	Never 1	N/A 0

12. Are the nostrils clean from food residues after chewing?

Always 5	Almost always 4	Sometimes 3	Almost never 2	Never 1	N/A 0

Form D

Food diary for dysphagics

By Antonio Amitrano and Elisa Matino

Date	With the aid of Operator Caregiver	Type of food or drink	Quantity	Cough	Discomfort during swallowing	Posture**
Breakfast	0 alone 0 with others		⊕	Yes No	Yes No	
Snack	0 alone 0 with others		⊕	Yes No	Yes No	
Lunch	0 alone 0 with others		⊕	Yes No	Yes No	
Snack	0 alone 0 with others		⊕	Yes No	Yes No	
Dinner	0 alone 0 with others		⊕	Yes No	Yes No	

** 1. The posture head was bent forward. 2. The posture head was flexed laterally. 3. The posture head was turned laterally. 4. The posture head was extended.

MIX
Papier aus verantwortungsvollen Quellen
Paper from responsible sources
FSC® C105338

If you have any concerns about our products,
you can contact us on
ProductSafety@springernature.com

In case Publisher is established outside the EU,
the EU authorized representative is:
Springer Nature Customer Service Center GmbH
Europaplatz 3, 69115 Heidelberg, Germany

Printed by Libri Plureos GmbH
in Hamburg, Germany